THIRD EDITION

Clinical Epidemiology

THE ESSENTIALS

THIRD EDITION

Clinical Epidemiology

THE ESSENTIALS

Robert H. Fletcher, M.D., M.Sc.

Professor
Department of Ambulatory Care and Prevention
Harvard Medical School and Harvard Community Health Plan
Department of Epidemiology, Harvard School of Public Health
Department of Medicine, Brigham and Women's Hospital
Boston, Massachusetts

Suzanne W. Fletcher, M.D., M.Sc.

Professor
Department of Ambulatory Care and Prevention
Harvard Medical School and Harvard Community Health Plan
Department of Epidemiology, Harvard School of Public Health
Department of Medicine, Brigham and Women's Hospital
Boston, Massachusetts

Edward H. Wagner, M.D., M.P.H.

Director, Center for Health Studies
Group Health Cooperative of Puget Sound
Professor of Health Services
University of Washington
Seattle, Washington

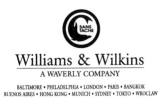

Williams & Wilkins

A WAVERLY COMPANY

BALTIMORE • PHILADELPHIA • LONDON • PARIS • BANGKOK
BUENOS AIRES • HONG KONG • MUNICH • SYDNEY • TOKYO • WROCLAW

Editor: Timothy S. Satterfield
Managing Editor: Crystal Taylor
Production Coordinator: Raymond E. Reter
Copy Editor: Candace B. Levy, Ph.D.
Designer: Norman W. Och
Illustration Planner: Mario Fernandez
Typesetter: Tapsco, Inc., Akron, Pennsylvania
Printer & Binder: Victor Graphics, Inc., Baltimore, Maryland

Copyright © 1996 Williams & Wilkins

351 West Camden Street
Baltimore, Maryland 21201-2436 USA

Rose Tree Corporate Center
1400 North Providence Road
Building II, Suite 5025
Media, Pennsylvania 19063-2043 USA

Accurate indications, adverse reactions and dosage schedules for drugs are provided in this book, but it is possible that they may change. The reader is urged to review the package information data of the manufacturers of the medications mentioned.

Printed in the United States of America

First Edition, 1982
Second Edition, 1988

Library of Congress Cataloging-in-Publication Data

Fletcher, Robert H.
  Clinical epidemiology: the essentials/Robert H. Fletcher,
Suzanne W. Fletcher, Edward H. Wagner. — 3rd ed.
    p. cm.
  Includes bibliographical references and index.
  ISBN 0-683-03269-0
  1. Clinical epidemiology. I. Wagner, Edward H. (Edward Harris),
1940-   . II. Title.
  [DNLM: 1. Epidemiologic Methods.   WA 950 F614c   1996]
RA652.2.C55F57 1996
614.4—dc20
DNLM/DLC
for Library of Congress   95-8382
                                                          CIP

The publishers have made every effort to trace the copyright holders for borrowed material. If they have inadvertently overlooked any, they will be pleased to make the necessary arrangements at the first opportunity.

95 96 97 98 99
1 2 3 4 5 6 7 8 9 10

PREFACE

Since the Second Edition was written in 1988, the pace of change in medicine has accelerated. Changes have brought greater recognition of the perspectives and methods of clinical epidemiology.

Countries throughout the world have, in their efforts to provide high-quality health care, experienced growing difficulties controlling the cost of care. The tension between demands for care and resources to provide it have increased the need for better information about clinical effectiveness in setting priorities. It has become clearer that not all clinical care is effective and that the outcomes of care are the best way of judging effectiveness. Variations in care among clinicians and regions, not explained by patients' needs and not accompanied by similar differences in outcomes, have raised questions about which practices are best. All these forces in modern society have increased the value of good clinical research and of those who can perform and interpret this research properly.

Phenomenal advances in understanding the biology of disease, especially at the molecular level, have also occurred. Discoveries in the laboratory increase the need for good patient-based research. They must be tested in patients before they can be accepted as clinically useful. Thus the two—laboratory science and clinical epidemiology—complement each other and are not alternatives or competitors.

Other aspects of medicine are timeless. Patients and physicians still face the same kinds of questions about diagnosis, prognosis, and treatment and still value the same outcomes: to relieve suffering, restore function, and prevent untimely death. We rely on the same basic strategies (cohort and case-control studies, randomized trials, and the like) to answer the questions. The inherent uncertainty of all clinical information, even that based on the best studies, persists.

In preparing the third edition of this text, we have tried to take into account the sweeping changes in medicine as well as what has not changed. We have left the basic structure of the book intact. We updated examples throughout in recognition that some diseases, such as AIDS, are new and others, such as peptic ulcer disease, are better understood.

We have tried to remember that the book's niche is as an introduction

v

to clinical epidemiology and to avoid pitching the presentation to our colleagues who already have a firm grasp of the basics. The presentation is meant to be as simple as the topic allows. However, the field is covered in somewhat greater depth on the belief that readers expect more of the book now than they did when the field was new.

This edition is still primarily for clinicians who wish to develop a systematic understanding of how the evidence base for patient care is developed and assessed. Researchers begin with many of the same basic needs. The text should be useful at any level of clinical training: from medical student to practicing clinician.

ACKNOWLEDGMENTS

We have been privileged to work with wonderful colleagues, many of them clinical epidemiologists. This edition of the text distills what we have learned from them and from our own efforts to use clinical epidemiology. Our teachers were the pioneers of this field: Archie Cochrane, John Cassell, Alvan Feinstein, David Sackett, Kerr White, and others. More recently we have learned from the many young physicians throughout the world who have believed in this way of thinking about health and medical care and have put their beliefs into practice. Many are members of distinct programs—such as the International Clinical Epidemiology Network (INCLEN) and the Robert Wood Johnson Clinical Scholars Program—but the number of groups has become too numerous to list each one here.

The Fletchers are especially grateful to the editorial staff of Annals of Internal Medicine, our colleagues during the four years we were Editors-in-Chief. Articles in peer-reviewed clinical journals are the written record of clinical epidemiology, and we learned a great deal from our efforts to select and improve manuscripts. We were able to begin work on the third edition of this text—a daunting task in the midst of a move from the American College of Physicians in Philadelphia to Boston—thanks to the hospitality of Drs. Steven Jones and Wendy Levinson of the Legacy Portland Hospitals, our hosts while we were on sabbatical in Oregon. Tom Inui invited us to our new academic home—the Department of Ambulatory Care and Prevention at Harvard Medical School and Harvard Community Health Plan—and provided all the fellowship and resources we needed to finish the writing.

Ed Wagner is grateful for having been given the privilege to explore the uses of clinical epidemiology in studying, planning, and improving care for the 0.5 million enrollees of Group Health Cooperative of Puget Sound. My contribution to this edition owes much to the stimulation and support of my colleagues at the Center for Health Studies, the Group Health delivery system, at the University of Washington.

This edition reflects all of our experiences from the time the three of us were together on the faculties of Medicine and Epidemiology at the University of North Carolina at Chapel Hill. Now, 13 years later and in different places, we appreciate more than ever the importance of the many colleagues who have helped us improve our understanding of clinical epidemiology and to express it more clearly.

CONTENTS

1

INTRODUCTION

A 51-year-old man asks to see you because of chest pain. He was well until 2 weeks ago, when he noticed tightness in the center of his chest while walking uphill. The tightness stopped after 2 to 3 min of rest. A similar discomfort occurred several times since then, sometimes during exercise and sometimes at rest. He smokes one pack of cigarettes per day and has been told that his blood pressure is "a little high." He is otherwise well and takes no medications. However, he is worried about his health, particularly about heart disease. A complete physical examination and resting electrocardiogram are normal except for a blood pressure of 150/96.

This patient is likely to have many questions. Am I sick? How sure are you? If I am sick, what is causing my illness? How will it affect me? What can be done about it? How much will it cost?

As the clinician caring for this patient, you must respond to these questions and use them to guide your course of action. Is the probability of serious, treatable disease high enough to proceed immediately beyond simple explanation and reassurance to diagnostic tests? How well do various tests distinguish among the possible causes of chest pain: angina pectoris, esophageal spasm, muscle strain, anxiety, and the like. For example, how helpful will an exercise electrocardiogram be in either confirming or ruling out coronary artery disease? If coronary disease is found, how long can the patient expect to have the pain? Will the condition shorten his life? How likely is it that other complications—congestive heart failure, myocardial infarction, or atherosclerotic disease of other organs—will occur? Will reduction of his risk factors for coronary disease—cigarette smoking and hypertension—reduce his risk? If medications control the pain, should the patient have coronary artery bypass surgery anyway?

Clinicians use various sources of information to answer these questions: their own experiences, the advice of their colleagues, and the medical literature. In general, they depend on past observations on other similar patients to predict what will happen to the patient at hand. The manner in which such observations are made and interpreted determines whether the conclusions they reach are valid, and thus how helpful the conclusions will be to patients.

Clinical Epidemiology

Clinical epidemiology is the science of making predictions about individual patients by counting clinical events in similar patients, using strong scientific methods for studies of groups of patients to ensure that the predictions are accurate. The purpose of clinical epidemiology is to develop and apply methods of clinical observation that will lead to valid conclusions by avoiding being misled by systematic error and chance. It is one important approach to obtaining the kind of information clinicians need to make good decisions in the care of patients.

CLINICAL MEDICINE AND EPIDEMIOLOGY

The term *clinical epidemiology* is derived from its two parent disciplines: clinical medicine and epidemiology. It is "clinical" because it seeks to answer clinical questions and to guide clinical decision making with the best available evidence. It is "epidemiologic" because many of the methods used to answer these questions have been developed by epidemiologists and because the care of individual patients is seen in the context of the larger population of which the patient is a member.

Clinical medicine and epidemiology began together (1). The founders of epidemiology were, for the most part, clinicians. It is only during this century that the two disciplines drifted apart, with separate schools, training, journals, and opportunities for employment. More recently, clinicians and epidemiologists have become increasingly aware that their fields interrelate and that each is limited without the other (2).

TRADITIONAL CLINICAL PERSPECTIVE

Clinicians have a special set of experiences and needs that has conditioned how they go about answering clinical questions. They are, by and large, concerned with individual patients. They know all of their patients personally; take their own histories; do their own physical examinations; and they accept an intense, personal responsibility for each patient's welfare. As a result, they tend to see what is distinctive about each one and are reluctant to lump patients into crude categories of risk, diagnosis, or treatment and to express patients' membership in these categories as a probability.

Because their work involves the care of a succession of individual patients and is demanding in its own right, clinicians tend to be less interested in patients who have not come to their attention because they are in some other medical setting or are not under medical care at all—even though these patients may be just as sick as the patients they see.

Clinical training has been oriented toward the mechanisms of disease through the study of biochemistry, anatomy, physiology, and other traditional basic sciences. These sciences powerfully influence medical students during their formative years and are a predominant force in clinical research and publications. This training fosters the belief that to understand the detailed processes of disease in individual patients is to understand medicine. The implication is that one can predict the course of disease and select appropriate treatments through knowledge of the mechanisms of disease.

THE NEED FOR AN ADDITIONAL "BASIC SCIENCE"

This traditional approach serves clinicians well under the right circumstances. It has identified many promising interventions—for example, vaccines, antimicrobial and vasoactive drugs, and synthetic hormones. It works well for correcting acid-base abnormalities and diagnosing and treating nerve compressions.

However, clinical predictions from knowledge of the biology of disease should ordinarily be considered hypotheses, to be tested by clinical research, about what might transpire in patients, because the mechanisms are only partly understood and many other factors in the genetic, physical, and social environments also affect outcome. For example, it has been shown, despite predictions to the contrary, that feeding diabetics simple sugars produces no worse metabolic effects than feeding them complex sugars, that some antiarrhythmic drugs actually cause arrhythmias, and that drugs that favorably affect the rheologic properties of sickle cells do not necessarily reduce the frequency and severity of sickle cell crises.

Personal experience is also a guide to clinical decision making. However, no one clinician can have enough direct experience to recognize all the subtle, long-term, interacting relationships that characterize most chronic diseases (see Chapter 6).

Therefore, for clinicians who intend to make up their own minds about the soundness of clinical information, some understanding of clinical epidemiology is as necessary as an understanding of anatomy, pathology, biochemistry, and pharmacology. Indeed, clinical epidemiology is one of the basic sciences, a foundation on which modern medicine is practiced.

ELEMENTS OF CLINICAL EPIDEMIOLOGY

Personal experience and medicine's basis in the biology of disease are both valuable, but they do not take into account some of the realities of clinical science, which might be summarized as follows:

- In most clinical situations the diagnosis, prognosis, and results of treatment are uncertain for individual patients and, therefore, must be expressed as probabilities

- Probability for an individual patient is best estimated by referring to past experience with groups of similar patients
- Because clinical observations are made on people who are free to do as they please and by clinicians with variable skills and biases, the observations may be affected by systematic errors that can cause misleading conclusions
- All observations, including clinical ones, are also influenced by the play of chance
- To avoid being mislead, clinicians should rely on observations that are based on sound scientific principles, including ways to reduce bias and estimate the role of chance.

THE SOCIAL CONTEXT OF CLINICAL EPIDEMIOLOGY

Important forces in modern society have accelerated the recognition of clinical epidemiologic methods and perspectives. The costs of medical care are rising beyond the point where even the most affluent societies are able to pay for all the care people want. Studies have shown wide variation in clinical practices without corresponding variation in outcomes of care, suggesting that not all common and expensive practices are useful. More rigorous methods of evaluating clinical evidence are being developed and are valued by decision makers. These observations have led to the consensus that clinical care should be based on the strongest possible research and should be judged by the outcomes it achieves at a cost society can afford. Also, individual patients are increasingly seen in relation to the larger group of which they are members, both to make accurate predictions about them and to assist in deciding which uses of limited medical resources do the most good for the most people.

Basic Principles

The basic purpose of clinical epidemiology is to foster methods of clinical observation and interpretation that lead to valid conclusions. The most credible answers to clinical questions are based on the following principles.

CLINICAL QUESTIONS

Types of questions addressed by clinical epidemiology are listed in Table 1.1. These are the same questions confronting the doctor and patient in the example presented at the beginning of this chapter. They are at issue in most doctor-patient encounters.

HEALTH OUTCOMES

The clinical events of primary interest in clinical epidemiology are the health outcomes of particular concern to patients and those caring for them (Table 1.2). They are the events doctors try to understand, predict, interpret, and change when caring for patients. An important distinction between

Table 1.1
Clinical Questions

Issue	Question
Abnormality	Is the patient sick or well?
Diagnosis	How accurate are tests used to diagnose disease?
Frequency	How often does a disease occur?
Risk	What factors are associated with an increased risk of disease?
Prognosis	What are the consequences of having a disease?
Treatment	How does treatment change the course of disease?
Prevention	Does an intervention on well people keep disease from arising? Does early detection and treatment improve the course of disease?
Cause	What conditions lead to disease? What are the pathogenetic mechanisms of disease?
Cost	How much will care for an illness cost?

Table 1.2
Outcomes of Disease (the Five Ds)[a]

Death	A bad outcome if untimely
Disease[b]	A set of symptoms, physical signs, and laboratory abnormalities
Discomfort	Symptoms such as pain, nausea, dyspnea, itching, and tinnitis
Disability	Impaired ability to go about usual activities at home, work, or recreation
Dissatisfaction	Emotional reaction to disease and its care, such as sadness or anger

[a] Perhaps a sixth D, destitution, belongs on this list because the financial cost of illness (for individual patients or society) is an important consequence of disease.
[b] Or illness, the patient's experience of disease.

clinical epidemiology and other medical sciences is that the events of interest in clinical epidemiology can be studied directly only in intact humans and not in animals or parts of humans, such as humeral transmitters, tissue cultures, cell membranes, and genetic sequences.

Biologic outcomes cannot properly be substituted for clinical ones without direct evidence that the two are related. Table 1.3 summarizes some biologic and clinical outcomes for the modern treatment of a patient with human immunodeficiency virus (HIV) infection. It is plausible, from what is known about the biology of HIV infection, that clinical outcomes such as opportunistic infections, Kaposi's sarcoma, and death would be better if an intervention reduced the decline in CD4+ cell counts and p34 antigen. However, there is evidence that these are incomplete markers of disease progression and response to treatment. It is too much to assume that patient outcomes would improve as a result of the intervention just because biologic markers do, because many other factors might determine the end result. Clinical decisions should, therefore, be based on direct evidence that clinical outcomes themselves are improved.

Table 1.3
Biologic and Clinical Outcomes: Treatment of Human Immunodeficiency Virus Infection

Disease	Interventions	Outcomes	
		Biologic	Clinical
HIV infection	Zidovudine DDI DDC	CD4+ counts p24 antigenemia Viremia	Opportunistic infections Quality of life Death
		Association known or assumed?	

NUMBERS AND PROBABILITY

Clinical science is at its strongest when measurements are quantitative, in part because numerical information allows better confirmation, more precise communication among clinicians and between clinicians and patients, and estimation of error. Clinical outcomes such as death, symptoms, or disability, can be counted and expressed as numbers. Although qualitative observation is also important in clinical medicine, it is not part of clinical epidemiology.

Individual patients will either experience a clinical outcome or not, but predicting whether or not an individual will do so is seldom exact. Rather, clinicians use the results of research to assign probabilities that the outcome will occur. The clinical epidemiologic approach accepts that clinical predictions are uncertain, but can be quantitated, by expressing predictions as probabilities—for example, that symptomatic coronary disease occurs in 1 in 100 middle-aged men per year, that cigarette smoking doubles one's risk of dying at all ages, and that exogenous estrogens reduce the risk of fractures from osteoporosis by half.

POPULATIONS AND SAMPLES

In general, *populations* are large groups of people in a defined setting (such as North Carolina) or with a certain characteristic (such as age >65 years). These include relatively unselected people in the community, the usual population for epidemiologic studies of cause, as well as groups of people selected because of their attendance in a clinic or hospital or because of a characteristic such as the presence or severity of disease, as is more often the case in clinical studies. Thus one speaks of the general population, a hospitalized population, or a population of patients with a specific disease.

A *sample* is a subset of a population and is selected from the population. Clinical research is ordinarily carried out on samples. One is interested in the characteristics of the defined population but must, for practical reasons, estimate them by describing a sample.

BIAS

Bias is "a process at any stage of inference tending to produce results that depart systematically from the true values" (3). Suppose, for example, that treatment A is found to work better than treatment B. What kinds of biases might have brought about this observation if it were not true? Perhaps A is given to healthier patients than is B; then the results could be due to the systematic difference in health between the groups of patients whether or not they were treated rather than to differences in the effectiveness of treatment. Or A might taste better than B so that patients take the drug more regularly. Or A might be a new, very popular drug and B an old one, so that researchers and patients are more inclined to think that the new drug works better whether or not it really does. All of these are examples of potential biases.

Observations on patients (whether for patient care or research) are particularly susceptible to bias. The process tends to be just plain untidy. As participants in a study, human beings have the disconcerting habit of doing as they please and not necessarily what would be required for producing scientifically rigorous answers. When researchers attempt to conduct an experiment with them, as one might in a laboratory, things tend to go wrong. Some people refuse to participate, while others drop out or choose another treatment. What is more, some of the most important things about humans—feelings, comfort, performance—are generally more difficult to measure than physical characteristics, such as blood pressure or serum sodium. Then, too, clinicians are inclined to believe that their therapies are successful. (Most patients would not want a physician who felt otherwise.) This attitude, so important in the practice of medicine, makes clinical observations particularly vulnerable to bias.

Although dozens of biases have been defined (4), most fall into one of three broad categories (Table 1.4).

Selection bias occurs when comparisons are made between groups of patients that differ in ways, other than the main factors under study, that affect

Table 1.4
Bias in Clinical Observation

- *Selection bias* occurs when comparisons are made between groups of patients that differ in determinants of outcome other than the one under study.
- *Measurement bias* occurs when the methods of measurement are dissimilar among groups of patients.
- *Confounding bias* occurs when two factors are associated ("travel together") and the effect of one is confused with or distorted by the effect of the other.

the outcome of the study. Groups of patients often differ in many ways—age, sex, severity of disease, the presence of other diseases, and the care they receive. If we compare the experience of two groups that differ on a specific characteristic of interest (for example, a treatment or a suspected cause of disease) but are dissimilar in these other ways and the differences are themselves related to outcome, the comparison is biased and little can be concluded about the independent effects of the characteristic of interest. In the example used earlier, selection bias would have occurred if patients given treatment A were healthier than those given treatment B.

Measurement bias occurs when the methods of measurement are consistently dissimilar in different groups of patients. An example of a potential measurement bias would be the use of information taken from medical records to determine if women on birth control pills were at greater risk for thromboembolism than those not on the Pill. Suppose a study were made comparing the frequency of oral contraceptive use among women admitted to a hospital because of thrombophlebitis and a group of women admitted for other reasons. It is entirely possible that women with thrombophlebitis, if aware of the reported association between estrogens and thrombotic events, might report use of oral contraceptives more completely than women without thrombophlebitis, because they had already heard of the association. For the same reasons, clinicians might obtain and record information about oral contraceptive use more completely for women with phlebitis than for those without it. If so, an association between oral contraceptives and thrombophlebitis might be observed because of the way in which the history of exposure was reported and not because there really is an association.

Confounding bias occurs when two factors are associated with each other, or "travel together," and the effect of one is confused with or distorted by the effect of the other. This could occur because of selection bias, by chance, or because the two really are associated in nature.

> *Example*   Is herpesvirus infection a cause of cervical cancer? It has been consistently observed that the prevalence of herpesvirus infection is higher in women with cervical cancer than in those without. However, both herpesvirus and a number of other infectious agents, themselves possible causes of cervical cancer, are transmitted by sexual contact. In particular, there is strong evidence that human papillomavirus infection leads to cervical cancer. Perhaps the higher prevalence of herpesvirus infection in women with cervical cancer is only a consequence of greater sexual activity and so is indirectly related to a true cause, which is also transmitted sexually (Fig. 1.1). To show that herpesvirus infection is associated with cervical cancer independently of other agents, it would be necessary to observe the effects of herpesvirus free of the other factors related to increased sexual activity (5).

Selection bias and confounding bias are not mutually exclusive. They are described separately, however, because they present problems at different

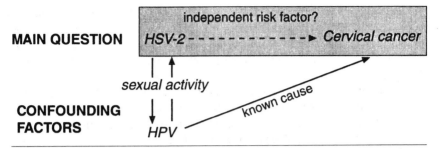

Figure 1.1. Confounding bias: Is herpesvirus 2 (HSV-2) a possible cause of cervical cancer? Only if its association with cervical cancer is independent of human papillomavirus (HPV) infection, known to be a cause of cervical cancer. Both viruses are related to increased sexual activity.

points in a clinical observation or study. Selection bias is at issue primarily when patients are chosen for observation, and so it is important in the design of a study. Confounding bias must be dealt with during analysis of the data, once the observations have been made.

Often in the same study more than one bias operates, as in the following hypothetical example.

> *Example*   A study was done to determine whether regular exercise lowers the risk of coronary heart disease (CHD). An exercise program was offered to employees of a plant, and the rate of subsequent coronary events was compared between employees who volunteered for the program and those who did not volunteer. Coronary events were determined by means of regular voluntary checkups, including a careful history, an electrocardiogram, and a review of routine health records. The group that exercised had lower rates of CHD. However, they also smoked cigarettes less.

In this example, selection bias could be present if volunteers for the exercise program were at lower risk for coronary disease even before the program began—for example, because they had lower serum lipids or less family history of coronary disease. Measurement bias might have occurred because the exercise group stood a better chance of having a coronary event detected, because more of them were examined routinely. Finally, the conclusion that exercise lowered the risk of coronary disease might be the result of a confounding bias if the association between exercise and coronary events in this particular study resulted from the fact that smoking cigarettes is a risk factor for coronary disease and the exercise group smoked less.

A potential for bias does not mean that bias is actually present in a particular study. For a researcher or reader to deal effectively with bias, it is first necessary to know where and how to look for it and what can be done about it. But one should not stop there. It is also necessary to determine whether bias is actually present and how large it is likely to be to decide whether it is important enough to change the conclusions of the study in a clinically meaningful way.

CHANCE

Observations about disease are ordinarily made on a sample of patients rather than all those with the disease in question. Observations on a sample of patients, even if unbiased, may misrepresent the situation in the population as a whole because of chance. However, if the observations were repeated on many such patient samples, results for the samples would vary about the true value. The divergence of an observation on a sample from the true population value, due to chance alone, is called *random variation*.

We are all familiar with chance as an explanation for why a coin does not come up heads exactly 50% of the time when it is flipped, say, 100 times. The same effect, random variation, applies when assessing the effects of treatments A and B, discussed earlier. Suppose all biases were removed from a study of the relative effects of the two treatments. Suppose, further, that the two treatments are, in reality, equally effective, each improving about 50% of the patients treated. Even so, because of chance alone a single study including small numbers of patients in each treatment group might easily find A improving a larger proportion of patients than B or vice versa.

Chance can affect all of the steps involved in clinical observations. In the assessment of treatments A and B, random variation occurs in the sampling of patients for the study, the selection of treatment groups, and the measurements made on the groups.

Unlike bias, which deflects values in one direction or another, random variation is as likely to result in observations above the true value as below it. As a consequence, the mean of many unbiased observations on samples tends to correspond to the true value in the population, even though the results of individual small samples may not.

Statistics can be used to estimate the probability of chance (random variation) accounting for clinical results. A knowledge of statistics can also help reduce that probability by allowing one to formulate a better design and analyses. However, random variation can never be totally eliminated, so chance should always be considered when assessing the results of clinical observations.

The relationship between bias and chance is illustrated in Figure 1.2. The measurement of diastolic blood pressure on a single patient is taken as an example. True blood pressure can be obtained by an intraarterial cannula, which is 80 mm Hg for this patient. But this method is not possible for routine measurements; blood pressure is ordinarily measured indi-

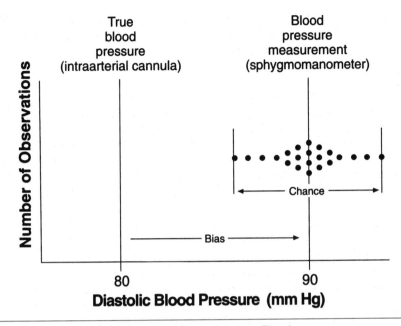

Figure 1.2. Relationship between bias and chance: Blood pressure measurements by intraarterial cannula and sphygmomanometer.

rectly, using a sphygmomanometer. The simpler instrument is prone to error, or deviations from the true value. In the figure, the error is represented by all of the sphygmomanometer readings falling to the right of the true value. The deviation of sphygmomanometer readings to the right (bias) may have several explanations—for example, a poorly calibrated sphygmomanometer, the wrong cuff size, or a deaf clinician. Bias could also result if different sounds were chosen to represent diastolic blood pressure. The usual end points—phase IV and phase V Korotkoff sounds—tend to be above and below the true diastolic pressure, respectively, and even that is unpredictable in obese people. Individual blood pressure readings are also subject to error because of random variation in measurement, as illustrated by the spread of the sphygmomanometer readings around the mean value (90 mm Hg).

The two sources of error—bias and chance—are not mutually exclusive. In most situations, both are present. The main reason for distinguishing between the two is that they are handled differently.

Bias can in theory be prevented by conducting clinical investigations properly or corrected through proper data analysis. If not eliminated, bias often can be detected by the discerning reader. Most of this book is about how to recognize, avoid, or minimize bias. Chance, on the other hand, cannot be eliminated, but its influence can be reduced by proper design of research, and the remaining error can be estimated by statistics. Statistics can also help remove the effects of known biases. However, no amount of statistical treatment can correct for unknown biases in data. Some statisticians would go so far as to suggest that statistics not be applied to data vulnerable to bias because of poor research design, for fear of giving false respectability to misleading work.

INTERNAL AND EXTERNAL VALIDITY

When making inferences about a population from observations on a sample, two fundamental questions arise (Fig. 1.3): First, are the conclusions of the research correct for the people in the sample? Second, if so, does the sample represent fairly the population of interest?

Internal validity is the degree to which the results of a study are correct for the sample of patients being studied. It is "internal" because it applies to the conditions of the particular group of patients being observed and not necessarily to others. The internal validity of clinical research is determined by how well the design, data collection, and analyses are carried out and is threatened by all of the biases and random variation discussed above. For a clinical observation to be useful, internal validity is a necessary but not sufficient condition.

External validity (generalizability) is the degree to which the results of an

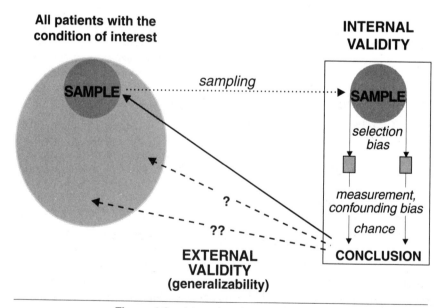

Figure 1.3. Internal and external validity.

observation hold true in other settings. For an individual physician, it is an answer to the question, "Assuming that the results of a study are true, do they apply to my patient as well?" Generalizability expresses the validity of assuming that patients in a study are comparable with other patients. An unimpeachable study, with high internal validity, may be totally misleading if its results are generalized to the wrong patients.

> *Example*   What is the risk that an abdominal aortic aneurysm will rupture? Clinicians seeing patients with aneurysms must have this information to make wise decisions about the need for elective surgical repair. The answer depends on which kinds of patients are described. Among patients with aneurysms <5 cm in diameter, above which surgery is commonly advised, those seen in referral centers have about a 10 times greater rate of rupture during 5 years of follow-up than those in the general population (Fig 1.4) (6). This may be because patients in centers are referred for symptoms or signs of impending rupture. If clinicians in office practice were to use the results of research from referral centers to predict rupture, they would greatly overestimate the risk and perhaps make the wrong decision about the need for elective surgical repair.

The generalizability of clinical observations, even those with high internal validity, is a matter of opinion about which reasonable people might disagree.

> *Example*   The Physician's Health Study showed that low-dose aspirin (325 mg every other day) prevented myocardial infarction in male physicians

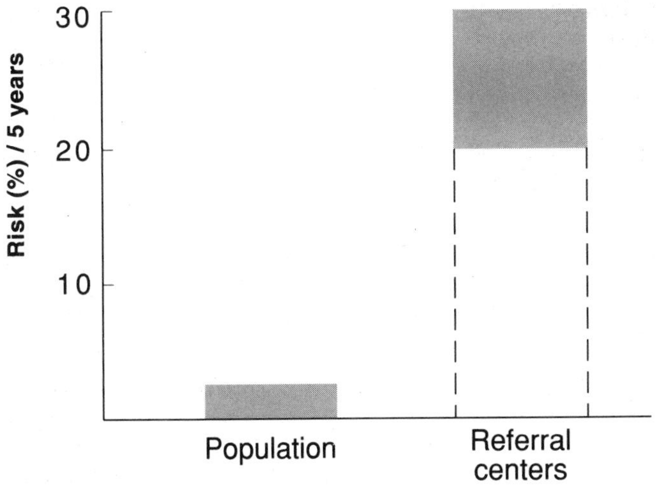

Figure 1.4.   Sampling bias: Range of risk of rupture (shaded area) in the next 5 years of abdominal aortic aneurysm (<5.0 cm in diameter) according to whether the patient is from the general population or a referral center (6).

without known coronary heart disease (7). The 11,037 physicians randomly assigned to take aspirin had a 44% lower rate of myocardial infarction than the 11,034 assigned to take placebo. The study was carefully conducted and used a strong research design; its findings have stood up well to criticisms. However, only healthy male physicians were in the study. When the results of the study were first released, clinicians had to decide whether it was justified to give aspirin to women, people with many risk factors, and patients who are already known to have coronary disease. Subsequently, reviews of evidence from all available studies have suggested that aspirin is also effective in these other groups of people (8).

Generalizability can rarely be dealt with satisfactorily in any one study. Even a defined, geographically based population is a biased sample of larger populations; for example, hospital patients are biased samples of county residents; counties, of states; states, of regions, and so on. Doing a study in many centers may improve generalizability, but does not settle the issue.

Usually, the best a researcher can do about generalizability is to ensure internal validity, have the study population fit the research question, and avoid studying groups so unusual that experience with them generalizes to few other patients. It then remains for other studies, in other settings, to extend generalizability.

Sampling bias has occurred when the sample of patients in a study is systematically different from those appropriate for the research question or the clinical use of the information. Because most clinical studies take place in medical centers and because patients in such centers usually overrepresent the serious end of the disease spectrum, sampling bias in clinical research tends to result in an exaggerated view of the serious nature of disease.

Uses of Clinical Epidemiology

Learning and applying clinical epidemiology adds time to an already busy clinician's schedule. What can he or she expect in return?

Understanding the strengths and weaknesses of clinical evidence, such as reports of research, gives intellectual satisfaction and confidence where there might otherwise be bewilderment and frustration. It can increase efficiency in acquiring sound information by allowing one to decide quickly, from basic principles, which articles or sources of clinical information are credible. During interaction with colleagues, it provides a sounder alternative to other ways of deciding where to invest belief in an assertion—the conviction, rhetoric, seniority, or specialty of the proponent. By relying on clinical epidemiology, clinicians of all backgrounds are on a more equal footing, all depending mainly on the interpretation of the same set of strong studies. Finally, clinical epidemiology gives clinicians a perspective on the extent to which their efforts, relative to other factors, such as the biology of disease and the physical and social environment, determine health outcomes, so that they can know what they can and cannot change.

For these reasons, we believe the time invested in learning clinical epidemiology is more than repaid.

Information and Decisions

The primary concerns of this book are the quality of clinical information and its correct interpretation. Making decisions is another matter. True, good decisions depend on good information; but they involve a great deal more as well, including value judgments and the weighing of competing risks and benefits.

In recent years, medical decision making has become a valued discipline in its own right. The field includes qualitative studies of how clinicians make decisions and how the process might be biased and can be improved. It also includes quantitative methods—decision analysis, cost-benefit analysis, and cost-effectiveness analysis—that present the decision-making process in an explicit way so its components and the consequences of assigning various probabilities and values to them can be examined.

Some aspects of decision analysis, such as evaluation of diagnostic tests, are included in this book. However, we have elected not to go deeply into medical decision making itself. Our justification is that decisions are only as good as the information used to make them, and we have found enough to say about the essentials of collecting and interpreting clinical information to fill a book. Readers who wish to delve more deeply into medical decision making can begin with some of the suggested readings listed at the end of this chapter.

Organization of the Book

This book is written for clinicians who wish to understand for themselves the validity of clinical observations to be able to judge the credibility of their own clinical observations, those of their colleagues, and research findings in the medical literature. We have not written primarily for those who do clinical research, but for all the rest who depend on it. However, we believe that the basic needs of those who do and those who use clinical research findings are similar.

In most textbooks of clinical medicine, information about disease is presented as answers to traditional clinical questions: diagnosis, clinical course, treatment, and the like. On the other hand, most books about clinical investigation are organized around research strategies such as clinical trials, surveys, and case-control studies. This way of organizing a book may serve those who perform clinical research, but it is awkward for clinicians.

Events	Natural History	Chapter Title

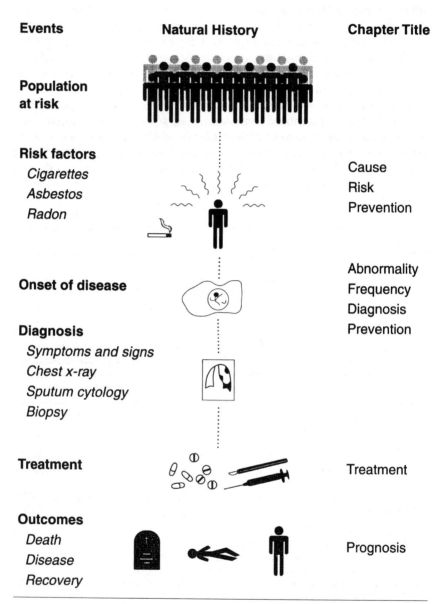

Events

Population at risk

Risk factors
Cigarettes
Asbestos
Radon

Onset of disease

Diagnosis
Symptoms and signs
Chest x-ray
Sputum cytology
Biopsy

Treatment

Outcomes
Death
Disease
Recovery

Chapter Title

Cause
Risk
Prevention

Abnormality
Frequency
Diagnosis
Prevention

Treatment

Prognosis

Figure 1.5. Organization of the book.

We have organized the book primarily according to the clinical questions encountered when doctors care for patients. Figure 1.5 illustrates how these questions correspond to the book chapters, taking lung cancer as an example. The questions relate to the entire natural history of disease, from the time people without lung cancer are first exposed to risk, through when some acquire the disease and emerge as patients, until the end results of disease are manifest.

In each chapter, we describe research strategies used to answer that chapter's clinical questions. Some strategies, such as cohort studies, are useful for answering several different kinds of clinical questions. For the purposes of presentation, we have discussed each strategy primarily in one chapter and simply referred to the discussion when the method is relevant to other questions in other chapters.

REFERENCES

1. White KL. Healing the schism. Epidemiology, medicine and public health. New York: Springer-Verlag, 1991.
2. Fletcher RH. Clinical medicine meets modern epidemiology—and both profit. Ann Epidemiol 1992;2:325–333.
3. Murphy EA. The logic of medicine. Baltimore: Johns Hopkins University Press, 1976.
4. Sackett DL. Bias in analytic research. J Chronic Dis 1979;32:51–63.
5. Jha PKS, Beral V, Peto J, Hack S, Hermon C, Deacon J, Mant D, Chilvers C, Vessey MP, Pike MC, Muller M, Gissmann L. Antibodies to human papillomavirus and to other genital infectious agents and invasive cervical cancer risk. Lancet 1993;341:1116–1118.
6. Ballard DJ. Abdominal aortic aneurysm [Letter]. New Engl J Med 1993;329:1275.
7. Steering Committee of the Physicians' Health Study Research Group. Final report on the aspirin component of the ongoing Physicians' Health Study. New Engl J Med 1989;321:129–135.
8. Antiplatelet Trialists' Collaboration. Collaborative overview of randomized trials of antiplatelet therapy—1. Prevention of death, myocardial infarction, and stroke by prolonged antiplatelet therapy in various categories of patients. Br Med J 1994;308:81–106.

SUGGESTED READINGS

Andersen B. Methodological errors in medical research. Boston: Blackwell Scientific Publications, 1990.

Eisenberg JM. Clinical economics. A guide to the economic analysis of clinical practices. JAMA 1989;262:2879–2886.

Facts, figures, and fallacies series

Jolley T. The glitter of the *t* table. Lancet 1993;342:27–29.

Victoria CG. What's the denominator? Lancet 1993;342:97–99.

Grisso JA. Making comparisons. Lancet 1993;342:157–160.

Datta M. You cannot exclude the explanation you haven't considered. Lancet 1993;342:345–347.

Mertens TE. Estimating the effects of misclassification. Lancet 1993;342:418–421.

Leon D. Failed or misleading adjustment for confounding. Lancet 1993;342:479–481.

Sitthi-amorn C, Poshachinda V. Bias. Lancet 1993;343:286–288.

Glynn JR. A question of attribution. Lancet 1993;342:530–532.

Carpenter LM. Is the study worth doing? Lancet 1993;343:221–223.

Feinstein AR. Clinical epidemiology. The architecture of clinical research. Philadelphia: WB Saunders, 1985.

Feinstein AR. Clinimetrics. New Haven, CT: Yale University Press, 1987.

Friedman GD. Primer of epidemiology. 4th ed. New York: McGraw-Hill, 1994.

Gehlbach SH. Interpreting the medical literature. 3rd ed. New York: McGraw-Hill, 1993.

Hennekins CH, Buring JE. Epidemiology in medicine. Boston: Little, Brown & Co, 1987.

Hulley SB, Cummings SR. Designing clinical research. An epidemiologic approach. Baltimore: Williams & Wilkins, 1988.

Jenicek M, Cleroux R. Epidemiologie clinique. Clinimetrie. St-Hyacinthe, Que., Canada: Edisem, 1985.

Kramer MS. Clinical epidemiology and biostatistics. A primer for clinical investigators and decision-makers. New York: Springer-Verlag, 1989.

Riegelman RK, Hirsch RP. Studying and study and testing a test. 2nd Ed. Boston: Little, Brown & Co, 1989.

Sackett DL, Haynes RB, Guyatt GH, Tugwell P. Clinical epidemiology. a basic science for clinical medicine. 2nd ed. Boston: Little, Brown & and Co, 1991.

Sox HC. Blatt MA, Higgins MC, Marton KI. Medical decision making. Stoneham, MA: Butterworth, 1988.

Users' guide to the medical literature series

Guyatt GH, Rennie D. Users' guides to the medical literature. JAMA 1993;270:2097-2098.

Oxman AD, Sackett DL, Guyatt GH. I. How to get started. JAMA 1993;270:2093-2095.

Guyatt GH, Sackett DL, Cook DJ. II. How to use and article about therapy or prevention. A. Are the results of the study valid? JAMA 1993;270:2598-2601.

Guyatt GH, Sackett DL, Cook DJ. II. How to use and article about therapy or prevention. B. What were the results and will they help me in caring for my patients? JAMA 1994;271:59-63.

Laupakis A, Wells G, Richardson S, Tugwell P. V. How to use an article about prognosis. JAMA 1994;272:234-237.

Jaeschke R, Guyatt G, Sackett DL. III. How to use and article about a diagnostic test. A. Are the results of the study valid? JAMA 1994;271:389-391.

Jaeschke R, Guyatt G, Sackett DL. III. How to use and article about a diagnostic test. B. What are the results and will they help me in caring for my patients? JAMA 1994;271:703-707.

Levine M, Walter S, Lee H, Haines T. Holbrook A, Moyer V. IV. How to use an article about harm. JAMA 1994;271:1615-1619.

Weiss NS. Clinical epidemiology. The study of the outcome of illness. New York: Oxford University Press, 1986.

White KL. Healing the schism. Epidemiology, medicine and the public's health. New York: Springer-Verlag, 1991.

2

ABNORMALITY

Clinicians spend a great deal of time distinguishing "normal" from "abnormal." When confronted with something grossly different from the usual, there is little difficulty telling the two apart. We all are familiar with pictures in textbooks of physical diagnosis showing massive hepatosplenomegaly, huge goiters, or severe changes of rheumatoid arthritis in the hand. We can take no particular pride in recognizing this degree of abnormality. More often, however, clinicians must make subtler distinctions between normal and abnormal. Is fleeting chest pain angina or inconsequential? Is a soft systolic heart sound a sign of valvular heart disease or an innocent murmur? Is a slightly elevated serum alkaline phosphatase evidence for liver disease, asymptomatic Paget's disease, or nothing important?

Decisions about what is abnormal are most difficult among relatively unselected patients, usually found outside of hospitals. When patients have already been selected for special attention, as is the case in most referral centers, it is usually clear that something is wrong. The tasks are then to refine the diagnosis and to treat the problem. In primary care settings, however, patients with subtle manifestations of disease are mixed with those with the everyday complaints of healthy people. It is not possible to pursue all of these complaints aggressively. Which of many patients with abdominal pain have self-limited gastroenteritis and which have early appendicitis? Which patients with sore throat and hoarseness have a garden variety pharyngitis and which the rare but potentially lethal *Haemophilus* epiglottitis? These are examples of how difficult, and important, distinguishing various kinds of abnormalities can be.

The point of distinguishing normal from abnormal is to separate out those clinical observations that should be considered for action from those that can be simply noted. Observations that are thought to be normal are usually described as "within normal limits," "unremarkable," or "noncontributory" and remain buried in the body of a medical record. The abnormal findings are set out in a problem list or under the heading "impressions" or "diagnoses" and are the basis for action.

Simply calling clinical findings normal or abnormal is undoubtedly crude and results in some misclassification. The justification for taking this approach is that it is often impractical or unnecessary to consider the raw data in all their detail. As Bertrand Russell put it, "To be perfectly intelligible one must be inaccurate, and to be perfectly accurate, one must be unintelligible." Physicians usually choose to err on the side of being intelligible—to themselves and others—even at the expense of some accuracy. Another reason for simplifying data is that each aspect of a clinician's work ends in a decision—to pursue evaluation or to wait, to select a treatment or reassure. Under these circumstances some sort of present/absent classification is necessary.

Table 2.1 is an example of how relatively simple expressions of abnormality are derived from more complex clinical data. On the left is a typical problem list, a statement of the patient's important medical problems. On the right are some of the data on which the decisions to call them problems are based. Conclusions from the data, represented by the problem list, are by no means noncontroversial. For example, the mean of the four diastolic blood pressure measurements is 94 mm Hg. Some might argue that this level of blood pressure does not justify the label "hypertension," because it is not particularly high and there are some disadvantages to telling patients they are sick and giving them pills. Others might consider the label fair, considering that this level of blood pressure is associated with an increased risk of cardiovascular disease and that the risk may be reduced by treatment. Although crude, the problem list serves as a basis for decisions—about diagnosis, prognosis, and treatment—and clinical

Table 2.1
Summarization of Clinical Data: A Patient's Problem List and the Data on Which It Is Based

Problem List	Raw Data
1. Hypertension	Several blood pressure readings (mm Hg): 170/102, 150/86, 166/92, 172/96
2. Diabetes mellitus	Glucose tolerance test:

	Time (h)	0	0.5	1	2
	Plasma glucose (mg/100 mL)	110	190	170	140

Problem List	Raw Data
3. Renal insufficiency	Serum chemistries: Creatinine 2.7 mg/100 mL Urea nitrogen 40 mg/100 mL Bicarbonate 18 mEq/L

decisions must be made, whether actively (by additional diagnostic tests and treatment) or passively (by no intervention).

This chapter describes some of the ways clinicians distinguish normal from abnormal. To do so, first it will be necessary to consider how biologic phenomena are measured, vary, and are summarized. Then it will be possible to consider how these data are used as a basis for value judgments about what is worth calling abnormal.

Clinical Measurement

Measurements of clinical phenomena yield three kinds of data: nominal, ordinal, and interval.

Nominal data occur in categories without any inherent order. Examples of nominal data are characteristics that are determined by a small set of genes (e.g., tissue antigens, sex, inborn errors of metabolism) or are dramatic, discrete events (e.g., death, dialysis, or surgery). These data can be placed in categories without much concern about misclassification. Nominal data that can be divided into two categories (e.g., present/absent, yes/no, alive/dead) are called *dichotomous.*

Ordinal data possess some inherent ordering or rank, such as small to large or good to bad, but the size of the intervals between categories cannot be specified. Some clinical examples include 1+ to 4+ leg edema, grades I to VI murmurs (heard only with special effort to audible with the stethoscope off the chest), and grades 1 to 5 muscle strength (no movement to normal strength)

For *interval* data, there is inherent order and the interval between successive values is equal, no matter where one is on the scale. There are two types of interval data. Continuous data can take on any value in a continuum. Examples include most serum chemistries, weight, blood pressure, and partial pressure of oxygen in arterial blood. The measurement and descriptions of continuous variables may in practice be confined to a limited number of points on the continuum, often integers, because the precision of the measurement, or its use, does not warrant greater detail. For example, a particular blood glucose reading may in fact be 193.2846573 . . . mg/100 mL but simply reported as 193 mg/100 mL. *Discrete* data, can take on only specific values and are expressed as counts. Examples of discrete data are the number of a woman's pregnancies and live births and the number of seizures a patient has per month.

It is for ordinal and numerical data that the following question arises: Where does normal leave off and abnormal begin? When, for example, does a large normal prostate become too large to be considered normal? Clinicians are free to choose any cutoff point. Some of the reasons for the choices will be considered later in this chapter.

Performance of Measurements

Whatever the type of measurement, its performance can be described in several ways, discussed below.

VALIDITY

As pointed out in Chapter 1, *validity* is the degree to which the data measure what they were intended to measure—that is, the results of a measurement correspond to the true state of the phenomenon being measured. Another word for validity is *accuracy*.

For clinical observations that can be measured by physical means, it is relatively easy to establish validity. The observed measurement is compared with some accepted standard. For example, serum sodium can be measured on an instrument recently calibrated against solutions made up with known concentrations of sodium. Clinical laboratory measurements are commonly subjected to extensive and repeated validity checks. For example, it is a national standard in the United States that blood glucose measurements be monitored for accuracy by comparing readings against high and low standards at the beginning of each day, before each technician begins a day, and after any changes in the techniques such as a new bottle of reagents or a new battery for the instrument. Similarly, the validity of a physical finding can be established by the results of surgery or an autopsy.

Other clinical measurements such as pain, nausea, dyspnea, depression, and fear cannot be verified physically. In clinical medicine, information about these phenomena is obtained by "taking a history." More formal and standardized approaches, used in clinical research, are structured interviews and questionnaires. Groups of individual questions (items) are designed to measure specific phenomena (such as symptoms, feelings, attitudes, knowledge, beliefs) called "constructs." Responses to questions concerning a construct are converted to numbers and grouped together to form "scales."

There are three general strategies for establishing the validity of measurements that cannot be directly verified by the physical senses.

Content validity is the extent to which a particular method of measurement includes all of the dimensions of the construct one intends to measure and nothing more. For example, a scale for measuring pain would have content validity if it included questions about aching, throbbing, burning, and stinging but not about pressure, itching, nausea, tingling, and the like.

Construct validity is present to the extent that the measurement is consistent with other measurements of the same phenomenon. For example, the researcher might show that responses to a scale measuring pain are related to other manifestations of the severity of pain such as sweating, moaning, writhing, and asking for pain medications.

Criterion validity is present to the extent that the measurements predict a directly observable phenomenon. For example, one might see if responses on a scale measuring pain bear a predictable relationship to pain of known severity: mild pain from minor abrasion, moderate pain from ordinary headache and peptic ulcer, and severe pain from renal colic.

Validity is not, as is often asserted, either present or absent; Rather, with these strategies one can build a case for or against the validity of a scale, under the conditions in which it is used, so as to convince others that the scale is more or less valid.

Because of their selection and training, physicians tend to prefer the kind of precise measurements the physical and biologic sciences afford, and they avoid or discount others, especially for research. Yet relief of symptoms and promoting satisfaction and a feeling of well-being are among the most important outcomes of care, central concerns of patients and doctors alike. To guide clinical decisions, research must include them, lest the "picture" of medicine painted by the research be distorted.

As Feinstein (1) put it:

> The term "hard" is usually applied to data that are reliable and preferably dimensional (e.g., laboratory data, demographic data, and financial costs). But clinical performance, convenience, anticipation, and familial data are "soft." They depend on subjective statements, usually expressed in words rather than numbers, by the people who are the observers and the observed.
>
> To avoid such soft data, the results of treatment are commonly restricted to laboratory information that can be objective, dimensional, and reliable—but it is also dehumanized. If we are told that the serum cholesterol is 230 mg per 100 ml, that the chest X-ray shows cardiac enlargement, and that the electrocardiogram has Q waves, we would not know whether the treated object was a dog or a person. If we were told that capacity at work was restored, that the medicine tasted good and was easy to take, and that the family was happy about the results, we would recognize a human set of responses.

RELIABILITY

Reliability is the extent to which repeated measurements of a stable phenomenon—by different people and instruments, at different times and places—get similar results. *Reproducibility* and *precision* are other words for this property.

The reliability of laboratory measurements is established by repeated measures—for example, of the same serum or tissue specimen—sometimes by different people and with different instruments. The reliability of symptoms can be established by showing that they are similarly described to different observers under different conditions.

The relationships between reliability and validity are shown in Figure 2.1. An instrument (laboratory apparatus or a questionnaire) used to collect

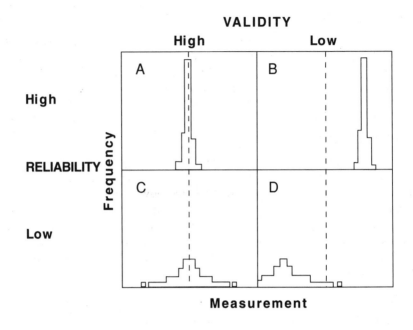

Figure 2.1.   Validity and reliability. *A*, High validity and high reliability. *B*, Low validity and high reliability. *C*, High validity and low reliability. *D*, Low validity and low reliability. The dotted lines represent the true values.

a large set of measurements can be valid (accurate) on the average but not be reliable, because the measures obtained are widely scattered about the true value. On the other hand, an instrument can be very reliable but be systematically off the mark (inaccurate). A single measurement with poor reliability has low validity because it is likely to be off the mark simply because of chance alone.

RANGE

An instrument may not register very low or high values of the thing being measured, limiting the information it conveys. Thus the "first-generation" method of measuring serum thyroid-stimulating hormone (TSH) was not useful for diagnosing hyperthyroidism or for precise titration of thyroxine administration because the method could not detect low levels of TSH. Similarly, the Activities of Daily Living scale (which measures people's ability at feeding, continence, transferring, going to the toilet, dressing, and bathing) does not measure inability to read, write, or play the piano—activities that might be very important to individual patients.

RESPONSIVENESS

An instrument is *responsive* to the extent that its results change as conditions change. For example, the New York Heart Association scale—classes I to IV (no symptoms, symptoms with slight and moderate exertion, and symptoms at rest)—is not sensitive to subtle changes in congestive heart failure, ones patients would value, whereas laboratory measurements of ejection fraction can detect changes too subtle for patients to notice.

INTERPRETABILITY

A disadvantage of scales based on questionnaires that is not generally shared by physical measurements is that the results may not have meaning to clinicians and patients. For example, just how bad is it to have a Zung depression scale value of 72? To overcome this disadvantage, researchers can "anchor" scale values to familiar phenomena—for example, by indicating that people with scores below 50 are considered normal and those with scores of 70 or over are severely or extremely depressed, requiring immediate care.

Variation

Clinical measurements of the same phenomenon can take on a range of values, depending on the circumstances in which they are made. To avoid erroneous conclusions from data, clinicians should be aware of the reasons for variation in a given situation and know which are likely to play a large part, a small part, or no part at all in what has been observed.

Overall variation is the sum of variation related to the act of measurement, biologic differences within individuals from time to time, and biologic differences from person to person (Table 2.2).

MEASUREMENT VARIATION

All observations are subject to variation because of the performance of the instruments and observers involved in making the measurement. The conditions of measurement can lead to a biased result (lack of validity) or

Table 2.2
Sources of Variation

Source	Definition
Measurement	
Instrument	The means of making the measurement
Observer	The person making the measurement
Biologic	
Within individuals	Changes in people with time and situation
Among individuals	Biologic differences from person to person

simply random error (lack of reliability). It is possible to reduce this source of variation by making measurements with great care and by following standard protocols. However, when measurements involve human judgment, rather than machines, variation can be particularly large and difficult to control.

> *Example* Fetal heart rate is often monitored by auscultation, which is subject to observer error. Electronic monitoring gives the true rate. Fetal heart rates that are unusually high or low are markers of fetal distress, suggesting a need for early delivery.
>
> Day et al. (2) compared fetal heart rates obtained by auscultation by hospital staff with rates obtained by electronic monitoring (Fig. 2.2). When the true fetal heart rate was in the normal range, rates by auscultation were evenly distributed about the true value, i.e., there was only random error. But when the true fetal heart rate was unusually high or low, rates by auscultation were biased toward normal. Low rates tended to be reported as higher than the true rates, and high rates as lower than the true rates.

This study illustrates both random and systematic errors in clinical observations. In this case, the bias toward normal rates might have arisen because the hospital staff hoped the fetus was well and were reluctant to undertake a major intervention based on their observation of an abnormally high or low heart rate.

Variations in measurements also arise because measurements are made on only a sample of the phenomenon being described, which may misrepresent the whole. Often the *sampling fraction* (the fraction of the whole that is included in the sample) is very small. For example, a liver biopsy represents only about 1/100,000 of the liver. Because such a small part of the whole is examined, there is room for considerable variation from one sample to another.

If measurements are made by several different methods (e.g., different laboratories, technicians, or instruments) some of the determinations may be unreliable and/or manifest systematic differences from the correct value, contributing to the spread of values obtained.

BIOLOGIC VARIATION

Variation also arises because of biologic changes within individuals over time. Most biologic phenomena change from moment to moment. A measurement at a point in time is a sample of measurements during a period of time and may not represent the usual value of these measurements.

> *Example* Clinicians estimate the frequency of ventricular premature depolarization (VPD) to help determine the need for and effectiveness of treatment. For practical reasons, they may do so by making relatively brief observations—perhaps feeling a pulse for 1 min or reviewing an electrocardiogram (a record of about 10 sec). However, the frequency of VPDs in a given patient varies over time. To obtain a larger sample of VPD rate, a portable (Holter) monitor is sometimes used. But monitoring even for extended periods of time can be misleading. Figure 2.3 shows observations on one patient with

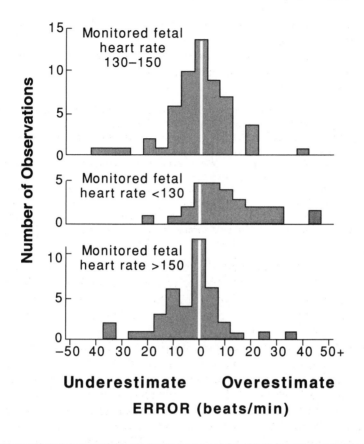

Figure 2.2. Observer variability. Error in reporting fetal heart rate according to whether the true rate, determined by electronic monitor, is within the normal range, low, or high. (Redrawn from Day E, Maddern L, Wood C. Auscultation of foetal heart rate: an assessment of its error and significance. Br Med J 1968;4:422–424.)

VPDs, similar to other patients studied (3). VPDs per hour varied from less than 20 to 380 during a 3-day period, according to day and time of day. The authors concluded: "To distinguish a reduction in VPD frequency attributable to therapeutic intervention rather than biologic or spontaneous variation alone required a greater than 83% reduction in VPD frequency if only two 24-hour monitoring periods were compared."

Variation also arises because of differences among people. Biologic differences among people predominate in many situations. For example, several studies have shown that high blood pressure on single, casual mea-

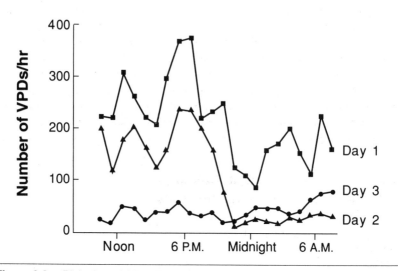

Figure 2.3.   Biologic variability. The number of ventricular premature depolarizations (VPDs) for one untreated patient on 3 consecutive days. (Redrawn from Morganroth J, Michelson EL, Horowitz LN, Josephson ME, Pearlman AS, Dunkman WB. Limitations of routine long-term electrocardiographic monitoring to assess ventricular ectopic frequency. Circulation 1978;58:408–414.)

surements, although subject to all other forms of variation, is related to subsequent cardiovascular disease.

TOTAL VARIATION

The several sources of variation are cumulative. Figure 2.4 illustrates this for the measurement of blood pressure. Variation from measurement contributes relatively little, although it covers as much as a 12 mm Hg range among various observers. On the other hand, each patient's blood pressure varies a great deal from moment to moment throughout the day, so that any single blood pressure reading might not represent the usual for that patient. Much of this variation is not random: blood pressure is generally higher when people are awake, excited, visiting physicians, or taking over-the-counter cold medications. Of course, we are most interested in knowing how an individual's blood pressure compares with that of his or her peers, especially if the blood pressure level is related to complications of hypertension and the effectiveness of treatment.

EFFECTS OF VARIATION

Another way of thinking about variation is in terms of its net effect on the validity and reliability of a measurement and what can be done about it.

Random variation—for example, by unstable instruments or many observers with various biases that tend to balance each other out—results on average in no net misrepresentation of the true state of a phenomenon if a set of measurements are made; individual measurements, however, may be misleading. Inaccuracy resulting from random variation can be reduced by taking a larger sample of what is being measured, for example, by counting more cells on a blood smear, examining a larger area of a urine sediment, or studying more patients. Also, the extent of random variation can be estimated by statistical methods (see Chapter 9).

On the other hand, biased results are systematically different from the true

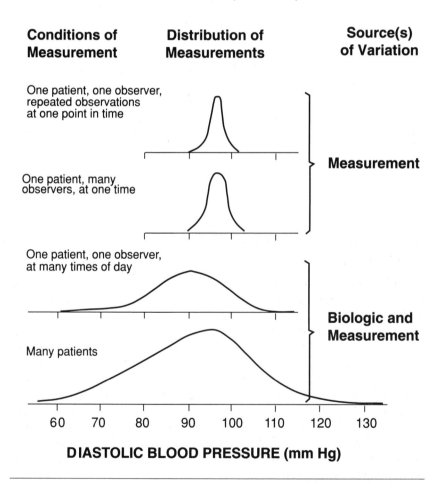

Conditions of Measurement

Distribution of Measurements

Source(s) of Variation

One patient, one observer, repeated observations at one point in time

One patient, many observers, at one time

Measurement

One patient, one observer, at many times of day

Many patients

Biologic and Measurement

60   70   80   90   100   110   120   130

DIASTOLIC BLOOD PRESSURE (mm Hg)

Figure 2.4.   Sources of variation. The measurement of diastolic (phase V) blood pressure. (Data from Fletcher RH and Fletcher SW; and Boe J, Humerfelt S, Wedervang F, Oecon C. The blood pressure in a population [Special Issue]. Acta Med Scand 1957;321:5–313.)

value, no matter how many times they are repeated. For example, when investigating a patient suspected of having an infiltrative liver disease (perhaps following up an elevated serum alkaline phosphatase) a single liver biopsy may be misleading, depending on how the lesions are distributed in the liver. If the lesion is a metastasis in the left lobe of the liver, a biopsy in the usual place (the right lobe) would miss it. On the other hand, a biopsy for miliary tuberculosis, which is represented by millions of small granulomata throughout the liver, would be inaccurate only through random variation. Similarly, all of the high values for VPDs shown in Figure 2.3 were recorded on the first day, and most of the low values on the third. The days were biased estimates of each other, because of variation in VPD rate from day to day.

Distributions

Data that are measured on interval scales are often presented as a figure, called a *frequency distribution*, showing the number (or proportion) of a defined group of people possessing the different values of the measurement (Fig. 2.5). Presenting interval data as a frequency distribution conveys the information in relatively fine detail.

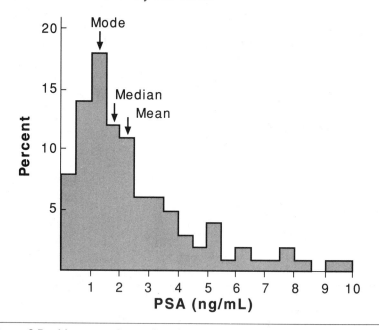

Figure 2.5. Measures of central tendency and dispersion. The distribution of prostate-specific antigen (PSA) levels in presumably normal men. (Data from Kane RA, Littrup PJ, Babaian R, Drago JR, Lee F, Chesley A, Murphy GP, Mettlin C. Prostate-specific antigen levels in 1695 men without evidence of prostate cancer. Cancer 1992;69:1201–1207.)

Table 2.3
Expressions of Central Tendency and Dispersion

Expression	Definition	Advantages	Disadvantages
Central Tendency			
Mean	Sum of values for observations ÷ Number of observations	Well suited for mathematical manipulation	Affected by extreme values
Median	The point where the number of observations above equals the number below	Not easily influenced by extreme values	Not well suited for mathematical manipulation
Mode	Most frequently occurring value	Simplicity of meaning	Sometimes there are no, or many, most frequent values
Dispersion			
Range	From lowest to highest value in a distribution	Includes all values	Greatly affected by extreme values
Standard deviation[a]	The absolute value of the average difference of individual values from the mean	Well suited for mathematical manipulation	For non-Gaussian distributions, does not describe a known proportion of the observations
Percentile, decile, quartile, etc.	The proportion of all observations falling between specified values	Describes the "unusualness" of a value without assumptions about the shape of a distribution	Not well suited for statistical manipulation

[a] $\sqrt{\dfrac{\Sigma(X - \bar{X})^2}{N - 1}}$

where X = each observation; $\bar{X}$ = mean of all observations; and N = number of observations.

DESCRIBING DISTRIBUTIONS

It is convenient to summarize distributions. Indeed, summarization is imperative if a large number of distributions are to be presented and compared.

Two basic properties of distributions are used to summarize them: *central tendency*, the middle of the distribution, and *dispersion*, how spread out the values are. Several ways of expressing central tendency and dispersion, along with their advantages and disadvantages, are summarized in Table 2.3 and illustrated in Figure 2.5.

ACTUAL DISTRIBUTIONS

The frequency distributions of four common blood tests (potassium, alkaline phosphatase, glucose, and hemoglobin) are shown in Figure 2.6. In general, most of the values appear near the middle, and except for the

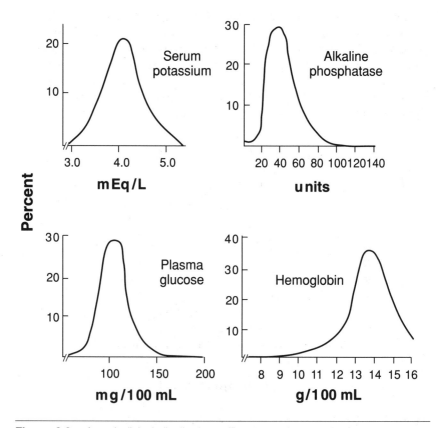

Figure 2.6. Actual clinical distributions. (Data from Martin HF, Gudzinowicz BJ, Fanger H. Normal values in clinical chemistry. New York: Marcel Dekker, 1975.)

central part of the curves, there are no "humps" or irregularities. The high and low ends of the distributions stretch out into tails, with the tail at one end often being more elongated than the tail at the other (i.e., the curves are "skewed" toward the long end). Whereas some of the distributions are skewed toward higher values, others are skewed toward lower values. In other words, all these distributions are unimodal, are roughly bell-shaped, and are not necessary symmetric; otherwise they do not resemble each other.

The distribution of values for many laboratory tests changes with characteristics of the patients such as age, sex, race, and nutrition. Figure 2.7 shows how the distribution of one such test, blood urea nitrogen (BUN), changes with age. A BUN of 25 mg/100 mL would be unusually high for a young person, but not particularly remarkable for an older person.

THE NORMAL DISTRIBUTION

Another kind of distribution, called the "normal" or Gaussian distribution, is sometimes assumed to approximate naturally occurring distributions, though it is based in statistical theory and has no necessary relationship to natural distributions. The normal curve describes the frequency distribution of repeated measurements of the same physical object by the same instrument. Dispersion of values represents random variation alone. A normal curve is shown in Figure 2.8. The curve is symmetrical and bell shaped. It has the

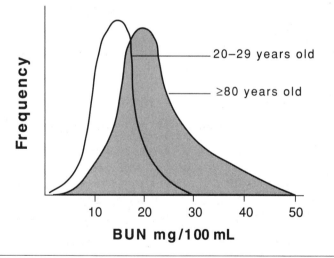

Figure 2.7. The distribution of clinical variables changes with age: BUN for people aged 20–29 versus those 80 or older. (Data from Martin HF, Gudzinowicz BJ, Fanger H. Normal values in clinical chemistry. New York: Marcel Dekker, 1975.)

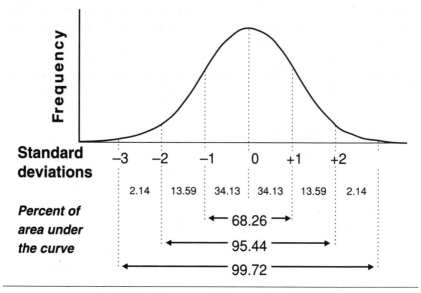

Figure 2.8. The normal (Gaussian) distribution.

mathematical property that about two-thirds of the observations fall within 1 standard deviation of the mean, and about 95% within 2 standard deviations.

Although clinical distributions often resemble a normal distribution the resemblance is superficial. As one statistician (4) put it:

> The experimental fact is that for most physiologic variables the distribution is smooth, unimodal, and skewed, and that mean ±2 standard deviations does not cut off the desired 95%. We have no mathematical, statistical, or other theorems that enable us to predict the shape of the distributions of physiologic measurements.

Whereas the normal distribution is derived from mathematical theory and reflects only random variation, many other sources of variation contribute to distributions of clinical measurements, especially biologic differences among people. Therefore, if distributions of clinical measurements resemble normal curves, it is largely by accident. Even so, it is often assumed, as a matter of convenience (because means and standard deviations are relatively easy to calculate and manipulate mathematically), that clinical measurements are "normally" distributed.

Criteria for Abnormality

It would be convenient if the frequency distributions of clinical measurements for normal and abnormal people were so different that these distributions could be used to distinguish two or more distinct populations.

This is the case for specific DNA and RNA sequences and antigens (Fig. 2.9A), which are either present or absent, although their clinical manifestations may not be so clear-cut.

However, most distributions of clinical variables are not easily divided into "normal" and "abnormal," because they are not inherently dichotomous and they do not display sharp breaks or two peaks that

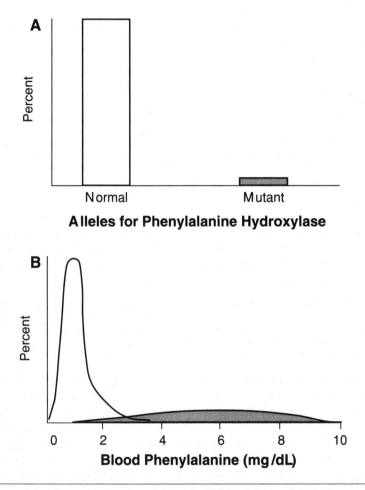

Alleles for Phenylalanine Hydroxylase

Blood Phenylalanine (mg/dL)

Figure 2.9. Screening for phenylketonuria (PKU) in infants: dichotomous and overlapping distributions of normal and abnormal. **A,** Alleles coding for phenylalanine hydroxylase are either normal or mutant. **B,** The distributions of blood phenylalanine levels in newborns with and without PKU overlap and are of greatly different magnitude. (The prevalence of PKU, actually about 1/10,000, is exaggerated so that its distribution can be seen in the figure.)

characterize normal and abnormal results. There are several reasons why this is so.

For many laboratory tests there are not even theoretical reasons for believing that distinct populations—well and diseased—exist. Disease is acquired by degrees, and so there is a smooth transition from low to high values with increasing degrees of dysfunction. Laboratory tests reflecting organ failure, such as serum creatinine for renal failure, behave in this way.

In other situations, well and diseased persons do in fact belong to separate populations, but when the two populations are mixed together they cannot be recognized as separate because values for the abnormals vary, they overlap those for normals, and there are few abnormals in the population.

> *Example* Phenylketonuria (PKU) is a disease characterized by progressive mental retardation in childhood. A variety of mutant alleles coding for phenylalanine hydroxylase results in dysfunction of the enzyme and, with a normal diet, accumulation of phenylalanine. The diagnosis, which becomes apparent in the first year of life, is confirmed by persistently high phenylalanine levels (several times the usual range) and low tyrosine levels in the blood.
>
> It is common practice to screen newborns for PKU with a blood test for phenylalanine a few days after birth, in time to treat before there is irreversible damage. However, the test misclassifies some infants, because at that age there is an overlap in the distributions of serum phenylalanine concentrations in infants with and without PKU and because infants with PKU make up only a small proportion of those screened, about 1/10,000 (Fig. 2.9B). Some newborns with PKU are in the normal range either because they have not yet ingested enough protein or because they have a combination of alleles associated with mild disease. Some children who are not destined to develop PKU have relatively high levels—for example, because their mothers have abnormal phenylalanine metabolism. The test is set to be positive at the lower end of the overlap between normal and abnormal levels, to detect most infants with the disease, even though only about 1 out of 5 infants with an abnormal screening test turns out to have PKU.

In unselected populations, the diseased patients often do not stand out because there are very few of them relative to normal people and because laboratory values for the diseased population overlap those for normals. The curve for diseased people is "swallowed up" by the larger curve for normal people. If, on the other hand, normal and diseased populations are mixed in more equal proportions—perhaps by selecting out for testing people with an unusually high likelihood of disease—then the resulting distribution could be truly bimodal. Even so, it would not be possible to choose a test value that clearly separates diseased and nondiseased persons (see Chapter 3).

If there is no sharp dividing line between normal and abnormal, and the clinician can choose where the line is placed, what ground rules should be used to decide? Three criteria have proven useful: being unusual, being sick, and being treatable. For a given measurement, the results of these approaches bear no necessary relation to each other, so that what might be considered abnormal using one criterion might be normal by another.

ABNORMAL = UNUSUAL

Normal often refers to the most frequently occurring or usual condition. Whatever occurs often is considered normal, and whatever occurs infrequently is abnormal. This is a statistical definition, based on the frequency of a characteristic in a defined population. Commonly, the reference population is made up of people without disease, but this need not be the case. For example, we may say that it is normal to have pain after surgery or for eczema to itch.

It is tempting to be more specific by defining what is unusual in mathematical terms. One commonly used way of establishing a cutoff point between normal and abnormal is to agree, somewhat arbitrarily, that all values beyond 2 standard deviations from the mean are abnormal. On the assumption that the distribution in question approximates a normal (Gaussian) distribution, 2.5% of observations would then appear in each tail of the distribution and be considered abnormal.

Of course, as already pointed out most biologic measurements are not normally distributed. So it is better to describe unusual values, whatever the proportion chosen, as a fraction (or percentile) of the actual distribution. In this way, it is possible to make a direct statement about how infrequent a value is without making assumptions about the shape of the distribution from which it came.

A statistical definition of normality is commonly used but there are several ways in which it can be ambiguous or misleading.

First, if all values beyond an arbitrary statistical limit, say the 95th percentile, were considered abnormal, then the prevalence of all diseases would be the same, 5%. This is inconsistent with our usual way of thinking about disease frequency.

Second, there is no general relationship between the degree of statistical unusualness and clinical disease. The relationship is specific to the disease in question. For some measurements, deviations from usual are associated with disease to an important degree only at quite extreme values, well beyond the 95th or even the 99th percentile.

Example   The World Health Organization (WHO) considers anemia to be present when hemoglobin (Hb) levels are below 12 g/100 mL in adult nonpregnant females. In a British survey of women aged 20–64, Hb was below 12 g/100 mL in 11% of 920 nonpregnant women, twice as many as would be expected if the criterion for abnormality were exceeding 2 standard deviations (5). But were the women with Hb levels below 12 g/100 mL "diseased" in any way because of their relatively low Hb? Two possibilities come to mind: The low Hb may be associated with symptoms or it may be a manifestation of serious underlying disease. Symptoms such as fatigue, dizziness, and irritability were not correlated with Hb level, at least for women whose Hb was above 8.0. Moreover, oral iron, given to women with Hb between 8.0 and 12.0, increased Hb by an average of 2.30 g/100 mL but did not lead to any greater improvement in symptoms than was experienced by women given placebo. As for serious underlying disease, it is true that occasionally low Hb may be a manifestation of cancer, chronic infection, or rheumatic diseases. But only a very small proportion of women with low Hb have these conditions.

Thus only at Hb levels below 8.0, which occurred in less than 1% of these women, might anemia be an important health problem.

Third, many laboratory tests are related to risk of disease over their entire range of values, from low to high. For serum cholesterol, there is an almost threefold increase in risk from the "low normal" to the "high normal" range.

Fourth, some extreme values are distinctly unusual but preferable to more usual ones. This is particularly true at the low end of some distributions. Who would not be pleased to have a serum creatinine of 0.4 mg/100 mL or a systolic blood pressure of 105 mm Hg? Both are unusually low but they represent better than average health or risk.

Finally, sometimes patients may have, for laboratory tests diagnostic of their disease, values in the usual range for healthy people, yet clearly be diseased. Examples include low pressure hydrocephalus, normal pressure glaucoma, and normocalcemic hyperparathyroidism.

ABNORMAL = ASSOCIATED WITH DISEASE

A sounder approach to distinguishing normal from abnormal is to call abnormal those observations that are regularly associated with disease, disability, or death, i.e., clinically meaningful departures from good health.

> *Example*   What is a "normal" alcohol (ethanol) intake? Several studies have shown a U-shaped relationship between alcohol intake and mortality: high death rates in abstainers, lower rates in moderate drinkers, and high rates in heavy drinkers (Fig. 2.10). It has been suggested that the lower death rates with increasing alcohol consumption, at the lower end of the curve, occur because alcohol raises high density lipoprotein levels, which protects against cardiovascular disease. Alternatively, when people become ill they reduce their alcohol consumption and this could explain the high rate of mortality associated with low alcohol intake (6). High death rates at high intake is less controversial: alcohol is a cause of several fatal diseases (heart disease, cancer, and stroke). The interpretation of the causes for the U-shaped curve determines whether it is as abnormal to abstain as it is to drink heavily.

ABNORMAL = TREATABLE

For some conditions, particularly those that are not troublesome in their own right (i.e., are asymptomatic), it is better to consider a measurement abnormal only if treatment of the condition represented by the measure-

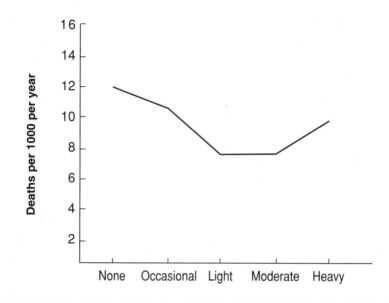

Figure 2.10. Abnormal as associated with disease. The relationship between alcohol consumption and mortality. (From Shaper AG, Wannamethee G, Walker M. Alcohol and mortality in British men: explaining the U-shaped curve. Lancet 1988;2:1267–1273.)

ment leads to a better outcome. This is because not everything that is associated with an increased risk can be successfully treated: the removal of the condition may not remove risk, either because the condition itself is not a cause of disease but is only related to a cause or because irreversible damage has already occurred. Also, to label people abnormal can cause adverse psychological effects that are not justified if treatment cannot improve the outlook.

What we consider treatable changes with time. At their best, therapeutic decisions are grounded on evidence from well-conducted clinical trials (Chapter 8). As new knowledge is acquired from the results of clinical trials, the level at which treatment is considered useful may change. For example, accumulating evidence for treating hypertension has changed the definition of what level is treatable. As more studies are conducted, successively lower levels of diastolic blood pressure have been shown to be worth treating.

Regression to the Mean

When clinicians encounter an unexpectedly abnormal test result, they tend to repeat the test. Often the second test result is closer to normal. Why does this happen? Should it be reassuring?

Patients selected because they represent an extreme value in a distribution can be expected, on the average, to have less extreme values on subsequent measurements. This occurs for purely statistical reasons, not because the patients have necessarily improved. The phenomenon is called *regression to the mean*.

Regression to the mean arises in the following way (Fig 2.11). People are first selected for inclusion in a study or for further diagnosis or treatment because their initial measurement for a trait fell beyond an arbitrarily selected cutoff point in the tail of a distribution of values for all the patients examined. Some of these people will remain above the cutoff point on subsequent measurements, because their true values are usually higher than average. But others who were found to have values above the cutoff point during the initial screening usually have lower values. They were selected only because they happened, through random variation, to have a high value at the time they were first measured. When the measurement is taken again, these people have lower values than they had during the first screening. This phenomenon tends to drag down the mean value of the subgroup originally found to have values above the cutoff point.

Thus patients who are singled out from others because of a laboratory test result that is unusually high or low can be expected, on average, to be closer to the center of the distribution if the test is repeated. Moreover, subsequent values are likely to be more accurate estimates of the true

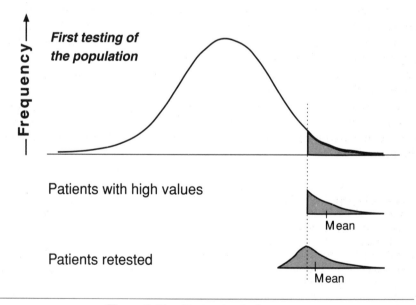

Figure 2.11. Regression to the mean.

value, which could be obtained if measurements were repeated for a particular patient many times. So the time-honored practice of repeating laboratory tests that are found to be abnormal and of considering the second one, which is often within normal limits, the correct one is not just wishful thinking. It has a sound theoretical basis. It also has an empirical basis. For example, it has been shown that half of serum T_4 tests found to be outside normal limits on screening were within normal limits when repeated (7). However, the more extreme the initial reading is, the less likely it is to be normal if it is repeated.

Summary

Clinical phenomena are measured on nominal, ordinal, and interval scales. Although many clinical observations fall on a continuum of values, for practical reasons they are often simplified into dichotomous (normal/abnormal) categories. Observations of clinical phenomena vary because of measurement error, differences in individuals from time to time, and differences among individuals. The performance of a method of measurement is characterized by validity (Does it measure what it intends to measure?), reliability (Do repeated measures of the same thing give the same result?), range, responsiveness, and interpretability.

Frequency distributions for clinical variables have different shapes, which can be summarized by describing their central tendency and dispersion.

Laboratory values from normal and abnormal people often overlap; because of this and the relatively low prevalence of abnormals, it is usually not possible to make a clean distinction between the two groups using the test result alone. Choice of a point at which normal ends and abnormal begins is arbitrary and is often related to one of three definitions of abnormality: statistically unusual, associated with disease, or treatable. If patients with extreme values of a test are selected and the test is repeated, the second set of values is likely to fall closer to the central (statistically normal) part of the frequency distribution, a phenomenon called regression to the mean.

REFERENCES

1. Feinstein AR. The need for humanized science in evaluating medication. Lancet 1972;2:421–423.
2. Day E, Maddern L, Wood C. Auscultation of foetal heart rate: an assessment of its error and significance. Br Med J 1968;4:422–424.
3. Morganroth J, Michelson EL, Horowitz LN, Josephson ME, Pearlman AS, Dunkman WB. Limitations of routine long-term electrocardiographic monitoring to assess ventricular ectopic frequency. Circulation 1978;58:408–414.
4. Elveback LR, Guillier CL, Keating FR. Health, normality, and the ghost of Gauss. JAMA 1970;211:69–75.

5. Elwood PC, Waters WE, Greene WJW, Sweetnam P. Symptoms and circulating hemoglobin level. J Chron Dis 1969;21:615–628.
6. Shaper AG, Wannamethee G, Walker M. Alcohol and mortality in British men: explaining the U-shaped curve. Lancet 1988;2:1267–1273.
7. Epstein KA, Schneiderman LJ, Bush JW, Zettner A. The "abnormal" screening serum thyroxine (T_4): analysis of physician response, outcome, cost and health and effectiveness. J Chron Dis 1981;34:175–190.

SUGGESTED READINGS

Department of Clinical Epidemiology and Biostatistics, McMaster University. Clinical disagreement I. How often it occurs and why. Can Med Assoc J 1980;123:499–504.

Department of Clinical Epidemiology and Biostatistics, McMaster University. Clinical disagreement II. How to avoid it and how to learn from one's mistakes. Can Med Assoc J 1980;123:613–617.

Feinstein AR. Clinical judgment. Baltimore: Williams & Wilkins, 1967.

Feinstein AR. Problems in measurement, clinical biostatistics. St. Louis: CV Mosby, 1977.

Feinstein AR. Clinimetrics. New Haven, CT: Yale University Press, 1987.

Koran LM. The reliability of clinical methods, data and judgment. N Engl J Med 1975;293:642–646, 695–701.

Mainland D. Remarks on clinical "norms." Clin Chem 1971;17:267–274.

Murphy EA. The logic of medicine. Baltimore: Johns Hopkins University Press, 1976

Guyatt GH, Feeny DH, Patrick DL. Measuring health-related quality of life. Ann Intern Med 1993;118:622–629.

3

DIAGNOSIS

Appearances to the mind are of four kinds. Things either are what they appear to be; or they neither are, nor appear to be; or they are, and do not appear to be; or they are not, yet appear to be. Rightly to aim in all these cases is the wise man's task

Epictetus, 2nd century A.D.

Clinicians devote a great deal of time to determining diagnoses for complaints or abnormalities presented by their patients. They arrive at the diagnoses after applying various diagnostic tests. Most competent clinicians use good judgment, a thorough knowledge of the literature, and a kind of rough-and-ready approach to how the information should be organized. However, there are also basic principles with which a clinician should be familiar when interpreting diagnostic tests. This chapter deals with those principles.

A *diagnostic test* is ordinarily taken to mean a test performed in a laboratory. But the principles discussed in this chapter apply equally well to clinical information obtained from history, physical examination, and imaging procedures. They also apply where a constellation of findings serves as a diagnostic test. Thus one might speak of the value of prodromal neurologic symptoms, headache, nausea, and vomiting in diagnosing classic migraine or of hemoptysis and weight loss in a cigarette smoker as indicators of lung cancer.

Simplifying Data

In Chapter 2, it was pointed out that clinical measurements, including data from diagnostic tests, are expressed on nominal, ordinal, or interval scales. Regardless of the kind of data produced by diagnostic tests, clinicians generally reduce the data to a simpler form to make them useful in practice. Most ordinal scales are examples of this simplification process. Obviously, heart murmurs can vary from very loud to inaudible. But trying to express subtle gradations in the intensity of murmurs is unnecessary for clinical decision making. A simple ordinal scale—grades I to VI—

serves just as well. More often, complex data are reduced to a simple dichotomy, e.g., present/absent, abnormal/normal, or diseased/well. This is particularly done when test results are used to decide on treatment. At any given point in time, therapeutic decisions are either/or decisions. Either treatment is begun or it is withheld.

The use of blood pressure data to decide about therapy is an example of how we simplify information for practical clinical purposes. Blood pressure is ordinarily measured to the nearest 2 mm Hg, i.e., on an interval scale. However, most hypertension treatment guidelines, such as those of the Joint National Committee on the Detection, Evaluation, and Treatment of Hypertension (1) and of most physicians, choose a particular level (e.g., 95 mm Hg diastolic pressure) at which to initiate drug treatment. In doing so, clinicians have transformed interval data into nominal (in this case, dichotomous) data. To take the example further, the Joint National Committee recommends that a physician choose a treatment plan according to whether the patient's diastolic blood pressure is "mildly elevated" (90–94 mm Hg), "moderately elevated" (95–114 mm Hg), or "severely elevated" (≥115 mm Hg), an ordinal scale.

The Accuracy of a Test Result

Establishing diagnoses is an imperfect process, resulting in a probability rather than a certainty of being right. In the past, the doctor's diagnostic certainty or uncertainty was expressed by using terms such as *rule out* or *possible* before a clinical diagnosis. Increasingly, the modern clinician expresses the likelihood that a patient has a disease by using a probability. That being the case, it behooves the clinician to become familiar with the mathematical relationships between the properties of diagnostic tests and the information they yield in various clinical situations. In many instances, understanding these issues will help the clinician resolve some uncertainty surrounding the use of diagnostic tests. In other situations, it may only increase understanding of the uncertainty. Occasionally, it may convince the clinician to increase his or her level of uncertainty.

A simple way of looking at the relationships between a test's results and the true diagnosis is shown in Figure 3.1. The test is considered to be either positive (abnormal) or negative (normal), and the disease is either present or absent. There are then four possible interpretations of the test results, two of which are correct and two wrong. The test has given the correct answer when it is positive in the presence of disease or negative in the absence of the disease. On the other hand, the test has been misleading if it is positive when the disease is absent (false positive) or negative when the disease is present (false negative).

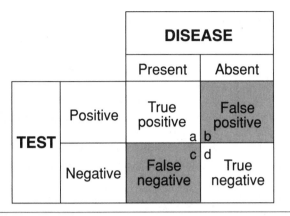

Figure 3.1. The relationship between a diagnostic test result and the occurrence of disease. There are two possibilities for the test result to be correct (true positive and true negative) and two possibilities for the result to be incorrect (false positive and false negative).

THE GOLD STANDARD

Assessment of the test's accuracy rests on its relationship to some way of knowing whether the disease is truly present or not—a sounder indication of the truth often referred to as the "gold standard." As it turns out, the gold standard is often elusive. Sometimes the standard of accuracy is itself a relatively simple and inexpensive test, such as a throat culture for group A β-hemolytic streptococcus to validate the clinical impression of strep throat or an antibody test for human immunodeficiency virus. However, this is usually not the case. More often, one must turn to relatively elaborate, expensive, or risky tests to be certain whether the disease is present or absent. Among these are biopsy, surgical exploration, and of course, autopsy.

For diseases that are not self-limited and ordinarily become overt in a matter of a few years after they are first suspected, the results of follow-up can serve as a gold standard. Most cancers and chronic, degenerative diseases fall into this category. For them, validation is possible even if on-the-spot confirmation of a test's performance is not feasible because the immediately available gold standard is too risky, involved, or expensive. Some care must be taken in deciding the length of the follow-up period, which must be long enough for the disease to manifest but not so long that cases can arise after the original testing.

Because it is almost always more costly and more dangerous to use these more accurate ways of establishing the truth, clinicians and patients prefer simpler tests to the rigorous gold standard, at least initially. Chest x-rays and sputum smears are used to determine the nature of pneumonia, rather than lung biopsy with examination of the diseased lung tissue. Similarly, electrocardiograms and serum enzymes are often used to establish the diagnosis of acute myocardial infarction, rather than catheterization or imaging procedures. The simpler tests are used as proxies for more elaborate but more accurate ways of establishing the presence of disease, with the understanding that some risk of misclassification results. This risk is justified by the safety and convenience of the simpler tests. But simpler tests are only useful when the risks of misclassification are known and found to be acceptably low. This requires sound data that compare their accuracy to an appropriate standard.

LACK OF INFORMATION ON NEGATIVE TESTS

The goal of all clinical studies describing the value of diagnostic tests should be to obtain data for all four of the cells shown in Figure 3.1. Without all these data, it is not possible to assess the risks of misclassification, the critical questions about the performance of the tests. Given that the goal is to fill in all four cells, it must be stated that sometimes this is difficult to do in the real world. It may be that an objective and valid means of establishing the diagnosis exists, but it is not available for the purposes of formally establishing the properties of a diagnostic test for ethical or practical reasons. Consider the situation in which most information about diagnostic tests is obtained. Published accounts come primarily from clinical, and not research, settings. Under these circumstances, physicians are using the test in the process of caring for patients. They feel justified in proceeding with more exhaustive evaluation, in the patient's best interest, only when preliminary diagnostic tests are positive. They are naturally reluctant to initiate an aggressive workup, with its associated risk and expense, when the test is negative. As a result, information on negative tests, whether true negative or false negative, tends to be much less complete in the medical literature.

This problem is illustrated by an influential study of the utility of the blood test that detects prostate specific antigen (PSA) in looking for prostate cancer (2). Patients with PSAs above a cutoff level were subjected to biopsy while patients with PSAs below the cutoff were not biopsied. The authors understandably were reluctant to subject men to an uncomfortable procedure without supporting evidence. As a result, the study leaves us unable to determine the false-negative rate for PSA screening.

LACK OF INFORMATION ON TEST RESULTS IN THE NONDISEASED

As discussed above, clinicians are understandably loath to perform elaborate testing on patients who do not have problems. An evaluation of a test's performance can be grossly misleading if the test is only applied to patients with the condition.

Example Magnetic resonance imaging (MRI) of the lumbar spine is frequently used in the evaluation of patients with low back pain. Many patients with back pain show herniated intervertebral disks on MRI, which often serves to explain the pain and guide treatment.

MRIs were performed on 98 asymptomatic volunteers (3). The studies were read by radiologists who did not know the symptom status of the patients. Bulging or protruding disks were found in nearly two-thirds of asymptomatic subjects, only slightly lower than the frequency of similar abnormality in patients with back pain. The authors concluded that such findings "may frequently be coincidental."

LACK OF OBJECTIVE STANDARDS FOR DISEASE

For some conditions, there are simply no hard-and-fast criteria for diagnosis. Angina pectoris is one of these. The clinical manifestations were described nearly a century ago, Yet there is still no better way to substantiate the presence of angina pectoris than a carefully taken history. Certainly, a great many objectively measurable phenomena are related to this clinical syndrome, for example, the presence of coronary artery stenoses seen on angiography, delayed perfusion on a thallium stress test, and characteristic abnormalities on electrocardiograms both at rest and with exercise. All are more commonly found in patients believed to have angina pectoris. But none is so closely tied to the clinical syndrome that it can serve as the standard by which the condition is considered present or absent.

Sometimes, usually in an effort to be "rigorous," circular reasoning is applied. The validity of a laboratory test is established by comparing its results to a clinical diagnosis, based on a careful history of symptoms and a physical examination. Once established, the test is then used to validate the clinical diagnosis gained from history and physical examination! An example would be the use of manometry to "confirm" irritable bowel syndrome, because the contraction pattern demonstrated by manometry and believed to be characteristic of irritable bowel was validated by clinical impression in the first place.

CONSEQUENCES OF IMPERFECT STANDARDS

Because of such difficulties as these, it is sometimes not possible for physicians in practice to find information on how well the tests they use compare with a thoroughly trustworthy standard. They must choose as their standard of validity another test that admittedly is imperfect but is considered the best available. This may force them into comparing one weak test against another, with one being taken as a standard of validity because it has had longer use or is considered superior by a consensus of experts. In doing so, a paradox may arise. If a new test is compared with an old (but inaccurate) standard test, the new test may seem worse even when it is actually better. For example, if the new test is more sensitive than the standard test, the additional patients identified by the new test would be considered false positives in relation to the old test. Just such a situation occurred in a comparison of real-time ultrasonography and oral cholecystography for the detection of gallstones (4). In five patients, ultrasound was positive for stones that were missed on an adequate cholecystogram. Two of the patients later underwent surgery and gallstones were found, so that for at least those two patients, the standard oral cholecystogram was actually less accurate than the newer real-time ultrasound. Similarly, if the new test is more often negative in patients who really do not have the disease, results for those patients will be considered false negatives compared with the old test. Thus, if an inaccurate standard of validity is used, a new test can perform no better than that standard and will seem inferior when it approximates the truth more closely.

Sensitivity and Specificity

Figure 3.2 summarizes some relationships between a diagnostic test and the actual presence of disease. It is an expansion of Figure 3.1, with the addition of some useful definitions. Most of the rest of this chapter deals

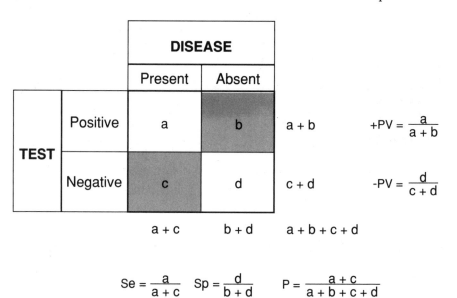

Figure 3.2.   Diagnostic test characteristics and definitions. Se = sensitivity; Sp = specificty; P = prevalence; PV = predictive value.

with these relationships in detail. Figure 3.3 illustrates these relationships. The diagnostic test is housestaff's clinical impression of whether patients complaining of pharyngitis have a group A β-hemolytic streptococcus infection or not, and the gold standard is a throat culture.

DEFINITIONS

As can be seen in Figure 3.2 *sensitivity* is defined as the proportion of people with the disease who have a positive test for the disease. A sensitive test will rarely miss people with the disease. *Specificity* is the proportion of people without the disease who have a negative test. A specific test will rarely misclassify people without the disease as diseased.

Applying these definitions to the pharyngitis example (Fig. 3.3), we see that 37 of the 149 patients with sore throats had positive cultures, and

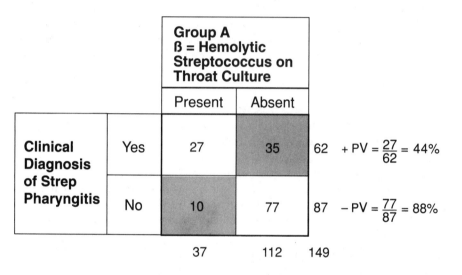

$$Se = \frac{27}{37} = 73\% \qquad Sp = \frac{77}{112} = 69\% \qquad P = \frac{37}{149} = 25\%$$

$$LR+ = \frac{\dfrac{27}{27 + 10}}{\dfrac{35}{35 + 77}} = 2.3 \qquad LR- = \frac{\dfrac{10}{10 + 27}}{\dfrac{77}{77 + 35}} = 0.39$$

Figure 3.3. The accuracy of the clinical diagnosis of streptococcal pharyngitis compared with the results of throat culture. (Data from Fletcher SW, Hamann C. Emergency room management of patients with sore throats in a teaching hospital; influence of non-physician factors. J Comm Health 1976;1:196–204.)

housestaff correctly diagnosed 27 of these—for a sensitivity of 73%. On the other hand, 112 patients had negative culture results; housestaff correctly withheld antibiotics from 77, for a specificity of 69%.

USES OF SENSITIVE TESTS

Clinicians should take the sensitivity and specificity of a diagnostic test into account when a test is selected. A sensitive test (i.e., one that is usually positive in the presence of disease) should be chosen when there is an important penalty for missing a disease. This would be so, for example, when there is reason to suspect a dangerous but treatable condition, such as tuberculosis, syphilis, or Hodgkin's disease. Sensitive tests are also helpful during the early stages of a diagnostic workup, when a great many possibilities are being considered, to reduce the number of possibilities. Diagnostic tests are used in these situations to rule out diseases, i.e., to establish that certain diseases are unlikely possibilities. For example, one might choose an HIV antibody test early in the evaluation of lung infiltrates and weight loss to rule out an AIDS-related infection. In sum, a sensitive test is most helpful to the clinician when the test result is negative.

USES OF SPECIFIC TESTS

Specific tests are useful to confirm (or "rule in") a diagnosis that has been suggested by other data. This is because a highly specific test is rarely positive in the absence of disease, i.e., it gives few false-positive results. Highly specific tests are particularly needed when false-positive results can harm the patient physically, emotionally, or financially. Thus, before patients are subjected to cancer chemotherapy, with all its attendant risks, emotional trauma, and financial costs, tissue diagnosis is generally required instead of relying on less specific tests. In sum, a specific test is most helpful when the test result is positive.

TRADE-OFFS BETWEEN SENSITIVITY AND SPECIFICITY

It is obviously desirable to have a test that is both highly sensitive and highly specific. Unfortunately, this is usually not possible. Instead, there is a trade-off between the sensitivity and specificity of a diagnostic test. This is true whenever clinical data take on a range of values. In those situations, the location of a *cut-off point*, the point on the continuum between normal and abnormal, is an arbitrary decision. As a consequence, for any given test result expressed on a continuous scale, one characteristic (e.g., sensitivity) can be increased only at the expense of the other (e.g., specificity). Table 3.1 demonstrates this interrelationship for the diagnosis of diabetes. If we require that a blood sugar taken 2 hr after eating be greater than 180 mg % to diagnose diabetes, all of the people diagnosed as "diabetic" would certainly have the disease, but many other people with diabetes would be missed using this extremely demanding definition

Table 3.1
Trade-Off between Sensitivity and Specificity when Diagnosing Diabetes[a]

Blood Sugar Level 2 hr after Eating (mg/100 mL)	Sensitivity (%)	Specificity (%)
70	98.6	8.8
80	97.1	25.5
90	94.3	47.6
100	88.6	69.8
110	85.7	84.1
120	71.4	92.5
130	64.3	96.9
140	57.1	99.4
150	50.0	99.6
160	47.1	99.8
170	42.9	100.0
180	38.6	100.0
190	34.3	100.0
200	27.1	100.0

[a] Public Health Service. Diabetes program guide. Publication no. 506. Washington, DC: U.S. Government Printing Office, 1960.

of the disease. The test would be very specific at the expense of sensitivity. At the other extreme, if anyone with a blood sugar of greater than 70 mg % were diagnosed as diabetic, very few people with the disease would be missed, but most normal people would be falsely labeled as having diabetes. The test would then be sensitive but nonspecific. There is no way, using a single blood sugar determination under standard conditions, that one can improve both the sensitivity and specificity of the test at the same time.

Another way to express the relationship between sensitivity and specificity for a given test is to construct a curve, called a *receiver operator characteristic (ROC) curve*. An ROC curve for the use of a single blood sugar determination to diagnose diabetes mellitus is illustrated in Figure 3.4. It is constructed by plotting the true-positive rate (sensitivity) against the false-positive rate (1-specificity) over a range of cut-off values. The values on the axes run from a probability of 0 to 1.0 (or, alternatively, from 0 to 100%). Figure 3.4 illustrates the dilemma created by the trade-off between sensitivity and specificity. A blood sugar cutoff point of 100 will miss only 11% of diabetics, but 30% of normals will be alarmed by a false-positive report. Raising the cutoff to 120 reduces false-positives to less than 10% of normals, but at the expense of missing nearly 30% of cases.

Tests that discriminate well crowd toward the upper left corner of the ROC curve; for them, as the sensitivity is progressively increased (the

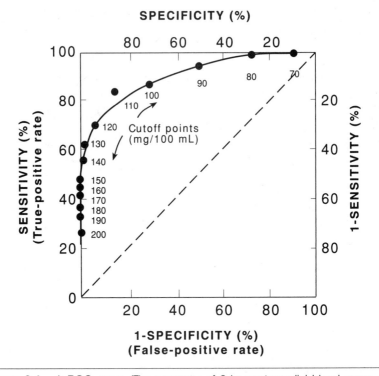

Figure 3.4. A ROC curve. The accuracy of 2-hr postprandial blood sugar as a diagnostic test for diabetes mellitus. (Data from Public Health Service. Diabetes program guide. Publication no. 506. Washington, DC: U.S. Government Printing Office, 1960.)

cutoff point is lowered) there is little or no loss in specificity until very high levels of sensitivity are achieved. Tests that perform less well have curves that fall closer to the diagonal running from lower left to upper right. The diagonal shows the relationship between true-positive and false-positive rates that would occur for a test yielding no information, e.g., if the clinician merely flipped a coin.

The ROC curve shows how severe the trade-off between sensitivity and specificity is for a test and can be used to help decide where the best cutoff point should be. Generally, the best cutoff point is at or near the "shoulder" of the ROC curve, unless there are clinical reasons for minimizing either false negatives or false positives.

ROC curves are particularly valuable ways of comparing alternative tests for the same diagnosis. The overall accuracy of a test can be described as the area under the ROC curve; the larger the area, the better the test.

Figure 3.5 compares the ROC curves for two questionnaire tests used to screen for alcoholism in elderly patients—the CAGE and the MAST (Michigan Alcoholism Screening Test) (5). The CAGE is both more sensitive and more specific than the MAST and includes a much larger area under its curve.

Obviously, tests that are both sensitive and specific are highly sought after and can be of enormous value. However, practicing clinicians rarely work with tests that are both highly sensitive and specific. So for the present, we must use other means for circumventing the trade-off between sensitivity and specificity. The most common way is to use the results of several tests together (as discussed below).

Establishing Sensitivity and Specificity

Not infrequently, a new diagnostic test is described in glowing terms when first introduced, only to be found wanting later when more experience with it has accumulated. Enthusiasm for the clinical value of serum

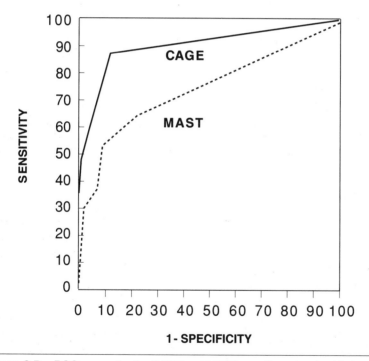

Figure 3.5. ROC curves for the CAGE and MAST questionnaires in elderly patients with and without alcoholism. (Redrawn from Jones TV, Lindsey BA, Yount P, Soltys R, Farani-Enayat B. Alcoholism screening questionnaires: are they valid in elderly medical outpatients? J Gen Intern Med 1993;8:674–678.)

carcinoembryonic antigen (CEA) waxed and then waned in this way. At first, CEA was considered a very promising means of diagnosing colon cancer. But subsequently CEA was shown to be increased in a wide variety of other conditions as well as in approximately 20% of smokers without cancer. This kind of confusion—initial enthusiasm followed by disappointment—arises not from any dishonesty on the part of early investigators or unfair skepticism by the medical community later. Rather, it is related to limitations in the methods by which the properties of the test were established in the first place. At the crudest level, the properties of a diagnostic test—sensitivity and specificity, for example—may be inaccurately described because an improper standard of validity has been chosen, as discussed previously. However, two other issues related to the selection of diseased and nondiseased patients can profoundly affect the determination of sensitivity and specificity as well. They are the spectrum of patients to which the test is applied and bias in judging the test's performance. A third problem that can lead to inaccurate estimates of sensitivity and specificity is chance.

SPECTRUM OF PATIENTS

Difficulties may arise when patients used to describe the test's properties are different from those to whom the test will be applied in clinical practice. Early reports often assess the test's value among people who are clearly diseased compared with people who are clearly not diseased, e.g., medical student volunteers. The test may be able to distinguish between these extremes very well.

Even patients with the disease in question can differ in severity, stage, or duration of the disease, and a test's sensitivity will tend to be higher in more severely affected patients.

> *Example* Figure 3.6 illustrates how the performance of the test CEA varies with the stage of colorectal cancer. CEA performs well for metastatic disease and poorly for localized cancer. Thus the sensitivity for "colorectal cancer" depends on the particular mix of stages of patients with disease used to describe the test, and its accuracy is more stable within stages (6).

Similarly, some kinds of people without disease, such as those in whom disease is suspected, may have other conditions that cause a positive test, thereby increasing the false-positive rate and decreasing specificity. For example, CEA is also elevated in many patients with ulcerative colitis or cirrhosis. If patients with these diseases were included in the nondiseased group when studying the performance of CEA for colorectal cancer, false positives would increase and the specificity of the test for cancer would fall.

In theory, the sensitivity and specificity of a test are said to be independent of the prevalence of diseased individuals in the sample in which the test is being evaluated. (Work with Figure 3.2 to confirm this for yourself.) In prac-

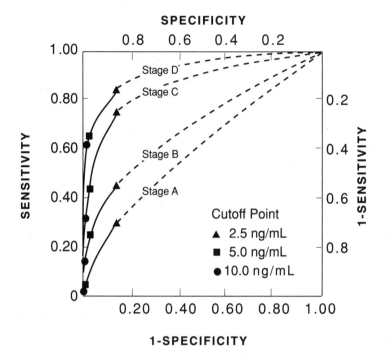

Figure 3.6.   ROC curve for CEA as a diagnostic test for colorectal cancer, according to stage of disease. The sensitivity and specificity of a test vary with the stage of disease. (Redrawn from Fletcher RH. Carcinoembryonic antigen. Ann Intern Med 1986;104:66–73.)

tice, however, several characteristics of patients, such as stage and severity of disease, may be related both to the sensitivity and specificity of a test and to the prevalence, because different kinds of patients are found in high- and low-prevalence situations. Using a test to screen for disease illustrates this point (see Chapter 8 for a fuller discussion of screening). Screening involves the use of the test in an asymptomatic population where the prevalence of the disease is generally low and the spectrum of disease favors earlier and less severe cases. In such situations, sensitivity tends to be lower and specificity higher than when the same test is applied to patients suspected of having the disease, more of whom have advanced disease.

BIAS

Sometimes the sensitivity and specificity of a test are not established independently of the means by which the true diagnosis is established, leading to a biased assessment of the test's properties. This may occur in several ways. As already pointed out, if the test is evaluated using data obtained during the course of a clinical evaluation of patients suspected of having the disease in question, a positive test may prompt the clinician to continue pursuing the diagnosis, increasing the likelihood that the disease will be found. On the other hand, a negative test may cause the clinician to abandon further testing, making it more likely that the disease, if present, will be missed.

In other situations, the test result may be part of the information used to establish the diagnosis, or conversely, the results of the test may be interpreted taking other clinical information or the final diagnosis into account. Radiologists are frequently subject to this kind of bias when they read x-rays. Because x-ray interpretation is somewhat subjective, it is easy to be influenced by the clinical information provided. All clinicians experience the situation of having x-rays overread because of a clinical impression, or conversely, of going back over old x-rays in which a finding was missed because a clinical event was not known at the time, and therefore, attention was not directed to the particular area in the x-ray. Because of these biases, some radiologists prefer to read x-rays twice, first without and then with the clinical information. All of these biases tend to increase the agreement between the test and the standard of validity. That is, they tend to make the test seem more useful than it actually is, as, for example, when an MRI of the lumbar spine shows a bulging disc in a patient with back pain (see earlier example in this chapter).

CHANCE

Values for sensitivity and specificity (or likelihood ratios, another characteristic of diagnostic tests, discussed below) are usually estimated from observations on relatively small samples of people with and without the disease of interest. Because of chance (random variation) in any one sample, particularly if it is small, the true sensitivity and specificity of the test can be misrepresented, even if there is no bias in the study. The particular values observed are compatible with a range of true values, typically characterized by the "95% confidence intervals"[1] (see Chapter 9). The width of this range of values defines the degree of precision of the estimates of sensitivity and specificity. Therefore, reported values for sensitivity and specificity should not be taken too literally if a small number of patients is studied.

---

[1] The 95% confidence interval of a proportion is easily estimated by the following formula, based on the binomial theorem:

$$p \pm 2\sqrt{\frac{p(1-p)}{N}}$$

where p is the observed proportion and N is the number of people observed. To be more nearly exact, multiply by 1.96.

Figure 3.7 shows how the precision of estimates of sensitivity increases as the number of people on which the estimate is based increases. In this particular example, the observed sensitivity of the diagnostic test is 75%. Figure 3.7 shows that if this estimate is based on only 10 patients, by chance alone the true sensitivity could be as low as 45% and as high as nearly 100%. When more patients are studied, the 95% confidence interval narrows, i.e., the precision of the estimate increases.

Predictive Value

As noted previously, sensitivity and specificity are properties of a test that are taken into account when a decision is made whether or not to order the test. But once the results of a diagnostic test are available, whether positive or negative, the sensitivity and specificity of the test are no longer relevant, because these values pertain to persons known to have or not to have the disease. But if one knew the disease status of the patient, it would not be necessary to order the test! For the clinician, the dilemma is to determine whether or not the patient has the disease, given the results of a test.

DEFINITIONS

The probability of disease, given the results of a test, is called the *predictive value* of the test (see Fig. 3.2). *Positive predictive value* is the probability of disease in a patient with a positive (abnormal) test result. *Negative pre-*

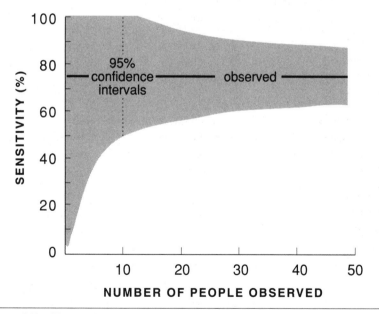

Figure 3.7. The precision of an estimate of sensitivity. The 95% confidence interval for an observed sensitivity of 75%, according to the number of people observed.

dictive value is the probability of *not* having the disease when the test result is negative (normal). Predictive value answers the question, "If my patient's test result is positive (negative) what are the chances that my patient does (does not) have the disease?" Predictive value is sometimes called *posterior* (or *posttest*) probability, the probability of disease *after* the test result is known. Figure 3.3 illustrates these concepts. Among the patients treated with antibiotics for streptococcal pharyngitis, less than half (44%) had the condition by culture (positive predictive value). The negative predictive value of the housestaff's diagnostic impressions was better; of the 87 patients thought not to have streptococcal pharyngitis, the impression was correct for 77 (88%).

Terms summarizing the overall value of a test have been described. One such term, *accuracy*, is the proportion of all test results, both positive and negative, that are correct. (For the pharyngitis example in Figure 3.3, the accuracy of the housestaff's diagnostic impressions was 70%.) The area under the ROC curve is another useful summary measure of the information provided by a test result. However, these summary measures are too crude to be useful clinically because specific information about the component parts—sensitivity, specificity, and predictive value at specific cutoff points—is lost when they are aggregated into a single index.

DETERMINANTS OF PREDICTIVE VALUE

The predictive value of a test is not a property of the test alone. It is determined by the sensitivity and specificity of the test and the prevalence of disease in the population being tested, where prevalence has its customary meaning—the proportion of persons in a defined population at a given point in time with the condition in question. Prevalence is also called *prior* (or *pretest*) probability, the probability of disease before the test result is known. (For a full discussion of prevalence, see Chapter 4.)

The mathematical formula relating sensitivity, specificity, and prevalence to positive predictive value is derived from Bayes's theorem of conditional probabilities:

$$\text{Positive predictive value} = \frac{\text{Sensitivity} \times \text{Prevalence}}{(\text{Sensitivity} \times \text{Prevalence}) + (1\text{-Specificity}) \times (1\text{-Prevalence})}$$

The more sensitive a test is, the better will be its negative predictive value (the more confident the clinician can be that a negative test result rules out the disease being sought). Conversely, the more specific the test is, the better will be its positive predictive value (the more confident the clinician can be that a positive test confirms or rules in the diagnosis being sought). Because predictive value is also influenced by prevalence, it is not independent of the setting in which the test is used. Positive results even for a very specific test, when applied to patients with a low likelihood of having the disease, will be largely false positives. Similarly, negative results, even for a very sensitive test, when applied to patients with a high chance of having the disease, are likely to be false negatives. In sum, the interpretation of a positive or negative diagnostic test result varies from setting to setting, according to the estimated prevalence of disease in the particular setting.

It is not intuitively obvious what prevalence has to do with an individual patient. For those who are skeptical it might help to consider how a test would perform at the extremes of prevalence. Remember that no matter how sensitive and specific a test might be (short of perfection), there will still be a small proportion of patients who are misclassified by it. Imagine a population in which no one has the disease. In such a group all positive results, even for a very specific test, will be false positives. Therefore, as the prevalence of disease in a population approaches zero, the positive predictive value of a test also approaches zero. Conversely, if everyone in a population tested has the disease, all negative results will be false negatives, even for a very sensitive test. As prevalence approaches 100%, negative predictive value approaches zero. Another way for the skeptic to convince himself or herself of these relationships is to work with Figure 3.2, holding sensitivity and specificity constant, changing prevalence, and calculating the resulting predictive values.

The effect of prevalence on positive predictive value, for a test at different but generally high levels of sensitivity and specificity, is illustrated in Figure 3.8. When the prevalence of disease in the population tested is relatively high—more than several percent—the test performs well. But at lower prevalences, the positive predictive value drops to nearly zero, and the test is virtually useless for diagnosing disease. As sensitivity and specificity fall, the influence of changes in prevalence on predictive value becomes more acute.

> *Example* The predictive value of PSA for diagnosing carcinoma of the prostate has been studied in various clinical situations, corresponding to different prevalences or prior probabilities. In older asymptomatic men, where the prevalence of prostatic carcinoma is estimated to be 6–12%, only about 15% of men with a PSA of 4 mg/dL or more actually had cancer. In higher risk men (with symptoms or a suspicious rectal exam), where the prevalence of prostatic carcinoma is 26%, 40% of men with positive PSAs had cancer (7). If PSA were used as a screening test in asymptomatic men, 5 or 6 healthy men would have to undergo additional tests, often including biopsy, to find one man with cancer. However, when there is a strong clinical suspicion of malignancy, nearly 50% of men with a positive test will have prostatic cancer.

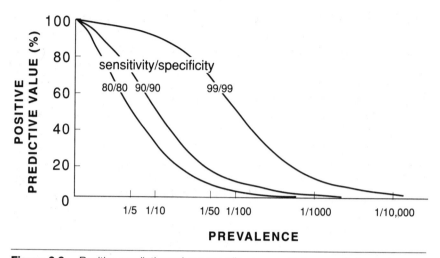

Figure 3.8.   Positive predictive value according to sensitivity, specificity, and prevalence of disease.

Current efforts to prevent transmission of acquired immunodeficiency syndrome (AIDS) through blood products is another example of the effect of disease prevalence on positive predictive value.

> *Example*   A blood test for antibodies to human immunodeficiency virus (HIV) is used to screen blood donors. At one cutoff point, the sensitivity is 97.8% and the specificity is 90.4%. In 1985, the positive predictive value of the test was estimated from the prevalence of infectious units to be no more than 1/10,000. Thus there would be 9,250 false-positive test results for every true-positive result (8). Almost 10,000 units would have to be discarded or investigated further to prevent one transfusion of contaminated blood. The authors concluded that, for this emotionally charged subject, "careful adherence to the principles of diagnostic test evaluation will avoid unrealistic expectations."
> But the situation changed. As the prevalence of HIV infection increased in the general population, the positive predictive value of the screening test improved. In a publication a year later, the prevalence of infected units among 67,190 tested was 25/10,000, and at similar levels of sensitivity and specificity, the positive predictive value would be 2.5%, much higher than a few years before (9).

ESTIMATING PREVALENCE

How can clinicians estimate the prevalence or probability of disease in a patient to determine the predictive value of a test result? There are several sources of information: the medical literature, local databases, and clinical judgment. Although the resulting estimate of prevalence is seldom very precise, error is not likely to be so great as to change clinical judgments that are based on the estimate. In any case, the process is bound to be more accurate than implicit judgment alone.

In general, prevalence is more important than sensitivity and specificity in determining predictive value (see Fig. 3.8). One reason why this is so is that prevalence commonly varies over a wider range. Prevalence of disease can vary from a fraction of a percent to near certainty in clinical settings, depending on the age, gender, risk factors, and clinical findings of the patient. Contrast the prevalence of liver disease in a healthy, young adult who uses no drugs, illicit or otherwise, and consumes only occasional alcohol, with that of a jaundiced intravenous drug user. By current standards, clinicians are not particularly interested in tests with sensitivities and specificities much below 50%, but if both sensitivity and specificity are 99%, the test is considered a great one. In other words, in practical terms sensitivity and specificity rarely vary more than twofold.

INCREASING THE PREVALENCE OF DISEASE

Considering the relationship between the predictive value of a test and prevalence, it is obviously to the physician's advantage to apply diagnostic tests to patients with an increased likelihood of having the disease being sought. In fact as Figure 3.8 shows, diagnostic tests are most helpful when the presence of disease is neither very likely nor very unlikely.

There are a variety of ways in which the probability of a disease can be increased before using a diagnostic test.

Referral Process

The referral process is one of the most common ways in which the probability of disease is increased. Referral to teaching hospital wards, clinics, and emergency departments increases the chance that significant disease will underlie patients' complaints. Therefore, relatively more aggressive use of diagnostic tests might be justified in these settings. In primary care practice, on the other hand, and particularly among patients without complaints, the chance of finding disease is considerably smaller, and tests should be used more sparingly.

> *Example* While practicing in a military clinic, one of the authors saw hundreds of people with headache, rarely ordered diagnostic tests, and never encountered a patient with a severe underlying cause of headache. (It is unlikely that important conditions were missed because the clinic was virtually the only source of medical care for these patients and prolonged follow-up was available.) However, during the first week back in a medical residency, a patient visiting the hospital's emergency department because of a headache similar to the ones managed in the military was found to have a cerebellar abscess!

Because clinicians may work at different extremes of the prevalence spectrum at various times in their clinical practices, they should bear in mind that the intensity of diagnostic evaluation may need to be adjusted to suit the specific situation.

Selected Demographic Groups

In a given setting, physicians can increase the yield of diagnostic tests by applying them to demographic groups known to be at higher risk for a disease. A man of 65 is 15 times more likely to have coronary artery disease as the cause of atypical chest pain than a woman of 30; thus the electrocardiographic stress test, a particular diagnostic test for coronary disease, is less useful in confirming the diagnosis in the younger woman than in the older man (10). Similarly, a sickle-cell test would obviously have a higher positive predictive value among blacks than among whites.

Specifics of the Clinical Situation

The specifics of the clinical situation are clearly the strongest influence on the decision to order tests. Symptoms, signs, and disease risk factors all raise or lower the probability of finding a disease. For example, a woman with chest pain is more likely to have coronary disease if she has typical angina and hypertension and she smokes. As a result, an abnormal electrocardiographic stress test is more likely to represent coronary disease in such a woman than in persons with nonspecific chest pain and no coronary risk factors.

The value of applying diagnostic tests to persons more likely to have a particular illness is intuitively obvious to most doctors. Nevertheless, with the increasing availability of diagnostic tests, it is easy to adopt a less selective approach when ordering tests. However, the less selective the approach, the lower the prevalence of the disease is likely to be and the lower will be the positive predictive value of the test.

The magnitude of this effect can be larger than most of us might think.

> *Example* Factors that influence the interpretation of an abnormal electrocardiographic stress test are illustrated in Figure 3.9. It shows that the positive predictive value for coronary artery disease (CAD) associated with an abnormal test can vary from 1.7 to 99.8%, depending on age, symptoms, and the degree of abnormality of the test. Thus an exercise test in an asymptomatic 35-year-old man showing 1 mm ST segment depression will be a false-positive test in more than 98% of cases. The same test result in a 60-year-old man with typical angina by history will be associated with coronary artery disease in more than 90% of cases (10).

Because of this effect, physicians must interpret similar test results differently in different clinical situations. A negative stress test in an asymptomatic 35-year-old man merely confirms the already low probability of coronary artery disease, but a positive test usually will be misleading if it is used to search for unsuspected disease, as has been done among joggers, airline pilots, and business executives. The opposite applies to the 65-

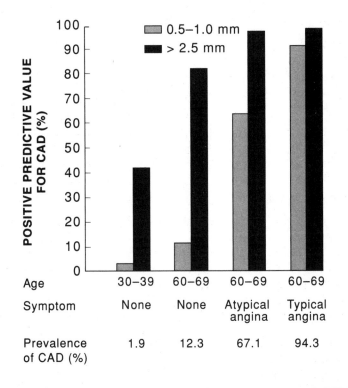

Age	30–39	60–69	60–69	60–69
Symptom	None	None	Atypical angina	Typical angina
Prevalence of CAD (%)	1.9	12.3	67.1	94.3

Figure 3.9.   Effect of disease prevalence on positive predictive value of a diagnostic test. Probability of coronary artery disease in men according to age, symptoms, and depression of ST segment on electrocardiogram. (Data from Diamond GA, Forrester JS. Analysis of probability as an aid in the clinical diagnosis of coronary artery disease. N Engl J Med 1979;300:1350–1358.)

year-old man with typical angina. In this case, the test may be helpful in confirming disease but not in excluding disease. The test is most useful in intermediate situations, in which prevalence is neither very high nor very low. For example, a 60-year-old man with atypical chest pain has a 67% chance of coronary artery disease before stress testing (see Fig. 3.9); but afterward, with greater than 2.5 mm ST segment depression, he has a 99% probability of coronary disease.

Because prevalence of disease is such a powerful determinant of how useful a diagnostic test will be, clinicians must consider the probability of disease before ordering a test. Until recently, clinicians relied on clinical observations and their experience to estimate the pretest probability of a disease. Research using large clinical computer data banks now provide quantitative estimates of the probability of disease, given various combinations of clinical findings (11).

IMPLICATIONS FOR THE MEDICAL LITERATURE

Published descriptions of diagnostic tests often include, in addition to sensitivity and specificity, some conclusions about the interpretation of a positive or negative test, i.e., predictive value. This is done, quite rightly, to provide information directly useful to clinicians. But the data for these publications are often gathered in university teaching hospitals where the prevalence of serious disease is relatively high. As a result, statements about predictive value in the medical literature may be misleading when the test is applied in less highly selected settings. What is worse, authors often compare the performance of a test in a number of patients known to have the disease and an equal number of patients without the disease. This is an efficient way to describe sensitivity and specificity. However, any reported positive predictive value from such studies means little because it has been determined for a group of patients in which the prevalence of disease was set by the investigators at 50%.

Likelihood Ratios

Likelihood ratios are an alternative way of describing the performance of a diagnostic test. They summarize the same kind of information as sensitivity and specificity and can be used to calculate the probability of disease after a positive or negative test.

ODDS

Because use of likelihood ratios depends on odds, to understand them it is first necessary to distinguish odds from probability. *Probability*—used to express sensitivity, specificity, and predictive value—is the proportion of people in whom a particular characteristic, such as a positive test, is present. *Odds*, on the other hand, is the ratio of two probabilities. Odds and probability contain the same information, but express it differently. The two can be interconverted using simple formulas:

$$\text{Odds} = \text{Probability of event} \div 1 - \text{Probability of event}$$

$$\text{Probability} = \text{Odds} \div 1 + \text{Odds}$$

These terms should be familiar to most readers because they are used in everyday conversation. For example, we may say that the odds are 4:1 that the Seattle Supersonics will win tonight or that they have an 80% probability of winning.

DEFINITIONS

The *likelihood ratio* for a particular value of a diagnostic test is defined as the probability of that test result in people with the disease divided by the probability of the result in people without disease. Likelihood ratios express how many times more (or less) likely a test result is to be found in diseased, compared with nondiseased, people. If a test is dichotomous (positive/negative) two types of likelihood ratios describe its ability to discriminate between diseased and nondiseased people: one is associated with a positive test and the other with a negative test (see Fig. 3.2).

In the pharyngitis example (see Fig. 3.3), the data can be used to calculate likelihood ratios for streptococcal pharyngitis in the presence of a positive or negative test (clinical diagnosis). A positive test is about 2.5 times more likely to be made in the presence of streptococcal pharyngitis than in the absence of it. If the clinicians believed streptococcal pharyngitis was not present, the likelihood ratio for this negative test was 0.39; the odds were about 1:2.6 that a negative clinical diagnosis would be made in the presence of streptococcal pharyngitis compared with the absence of the disease.

USES OF LIKELIHOOD RATIOS

Pretest probability (prevalence) can be converted to pretest odds using the formula presented earlier. Likelihood ratios can then be used to convert pretest odds to posttest odds, by means of the following formula:

$$\text{Pretest odds} \times \text{Likelihood ratio} = \text{Posttest odds}$$

Posttest odds can, in turn, be converted back to a probability, using the formula described earlier in this chapter. In these relationships, pretest odds contains the same information as prior probability (prevalence), likelihood ratios the same as sensitivity/specificity, and posttest odds the same as positive predictive value (posttest probability).

The main advantage of likelihood ratios is that they make it easier for us to go beyond the simple and clumsy classification of a test result as either abnormal or normal, as is usually done when describing the accuracy of a diagnostic test only in terms of sensitivity and specificity at a single cutoff point. Obviously, disease is more likely in the presence of an extremely abnormal test result than it is for a marginal one. With likelihood ratios, it is possible to summarize the information contained in a test result at different levels. One can define likelihood ratios for any number of test results, over the entire range of possible values. In this way, information represented by the degree of abnormality, rather than the crude presence or absence of it, is not discarded. In computing likelihood ratios across a range of test results, sensitivity refers to the ability of that particular test result to identify people with the disease, not individuals with that result or worse. The same is true for the calculation of specificity.

Thus likelihood ratios can accommodate the common and reasonable clinical practice of putting more weight on extremely high (or low) test results than on borderline ones when estimating the probability (or odds) that a particular disease is present.

Example How accurate is serum thyroxine (T_4) alone as a test for hypothyroidism? This question was addressed in a study of 120 ambulatory general medical patients suspected of having hypothyroidism (12). Patients were diagnosed as being hypothyroid if serum thyrotropin (TSH) was elevated and if subsequent evaluations, including other thyroid tests and response to treatment, were consistent with hypothyroidism. The authors studied the initial T_4 level in 27 patients with hypothyroidism and 93 patients who were found not to have it to determine how accurately the simple test alone might have diagnosed hypothyroidism.

As expected, likelihood ratios for hypothyroidism were highest for low levels of T_4 and lowest for high levels (Table 3.2). The lowest values in the distribution of T_4s (<4.0 μg/dL) were only seen in patients with hypothyroidism, i.e., these levels ruled in the diagnosis. The highest levels (>8.0 μg/dL) were not seen in patients with hypothyroidism, i.e., the presence of these levels ruled out the disease.

The authors concluded that "it may be possible to achieve cost savings without loss of diagnostic accuracy by using a single total T_4 measurement for the initial evaluation of suspected hypothyroidism in selected patients."

The likelihood ratio has several other advantages over sensitivity and specificity as a description of test performance. The information contributed by the test is summarized in one number instead of two. The calculations necessary for obtaining posttest odds from pretest odds are easy.

Table 3.2
Distribution of Values for Serum Thyroxine in Hypothyroid and Normal Patients, with Calculation of Likelihood Ratios[a]

Total Serum Thyroxine (μg/dL)	Patients with Test Result		Likelihood Ratio
	Hypothyroid (number, percent)	Normal (number, percent)	
<1.1	2 (7.4)		↑
1.1–2.0	3 (11.1)		Ruled in
2.1–3.0	1 (3.7)		
3.1–4.0	8 (29.6)		↓
4.1–5.0	4 (14.8)	1 (1.1)	13.8
5.1–6.0	4 (14.8)	6 (6.5)	2.3
6.1–7.0	3 (11.1)	11 (11.8)	.9
7.1–8.0	2 (7.4)	19 (20.4)	.4
8.1–9.0		17 (18.3)	↑
9.1–10		20 (21.5)	
10.1–11		11 (11.8)	Ruled out
11.1–12		4 (4.3)	
>12		4 (4.3)	↓
Total	27 (100)	93 (100)	

[a] From Goldstein BJ, Mushlin AI. Use of a single thyroxine test to evaluate ambulatory medical patients for suspected hypothyroidism. J Gen Intern Med 1987;2:20–24.

Also, likelihood ratios are particularly well suited for describing the overall probability of disease when a series of diagnostic tests is used (see below). Likelihood ratios (LR) also have disadvantages. One must use odds, not probabilities, and most of us find thinking in terms of odds more difficult than probabilities. Also, the conversion from probability to odds and back requires math or the use of a nomogram, which partly offsets the simplicity of calculating posttest odds using LRs. Finally, for tests with a range of results, LRs use measures of sensitivity and specificity that are different from those usually described.

Multiple Tests

Because clinicians commonly use imperfect diagnostic tests, with less than 100% sensitivity and specificity and intermediate likelihood ratios, a single test frequently results in a probability of disease that is neither very high nor very low, e.g., somewhere between 10% and 90%. Usually it is not acceptable to stop the diagnostic process at such a point. Would a physician or patient be satisfied with the conclusion that the patient has even a 20% chance of having carcinoma of the colon? Or that an asymptomatic 35-year-old man with 2.5 mm ST segment depression on a stress test has a 42% chance of coronary artery disease (see Fig. 3.9)? Even for less deadly diseases, such as hypothyroidism, tests with intermediate posttest probabilities are of little help. The physician is ordinarily bound to raise or lower the probability of disease substantially in such situations—unless, of course, the diagnostic possibilities are all trivial, nothing could be done about the result, or the risk of proceeding further is prohibitive. When these exceptions do not apply, the doctor will want to proceed with further tests.

When multiple tests are performed and all are positive or all are negative, the interpretation is straightforward. All too often, however, some are positive and others are negative. Interpretation is then more complicated. This section discusses the principles by which multiple tests are applied and interpreted.

Multiple tests can be applied in two general ways (Fig. 3.10). They can be used in *parallel* (i.e., all at once), and a positive result of any test is considered evidence for disease. Or they can be done *serially* (i.e., consecutively), based on the results of the previous test. For serial testing, all tests must give a positive result for the diagnosis to be made, because the diagnostic process is stopped when a negative result is obtained.

PARALLEL TESTS

Physicians usually order tests in parallel when rapid assessment is necessary, as in hospitalized or emergency patients, or for ambulatory patients who cannot return easily because they have come from a long distance for evaluation.

STRATEGY	SEQUENCE OF EVENTS	CONSEQUENCES

Serial testing

Test A *and* test B *and* test C are positive

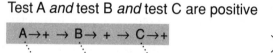

↓Sensitivity

↑Specificity

Parallel testing

Test A *or* test B *or* test C is positive

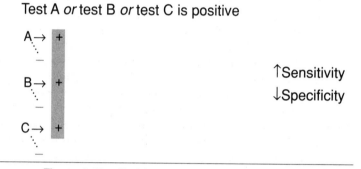

↑Sensitivity

↓Specificity

Figure 3.10. Serial and parallel testing.

Multiple tests in parallel generally increase the sensitivity and, therefore, the negative predictive value for a given disease prevalence above those of each individual test. On the other hand, specificity and positive predictive value are lowered. That is, disease is less likely to be missed (parallel testing is probably one reason referral centers seem to diagnose disease that local physicians miss), but false-positive diagnoses are also more likely to be made (thus the propensity for overdiagnosing in such centers as well). The degree to which sensitivity and negative predictive value increases depends on the extent to which the tests identify patients with the disease missed by the other tests used. For example, if two tests are used in parallel with 60 and 80% sensitivities, the sensitivity of the parallel testing will be only 80% if the better test identifies all the cases found by the less sensitive test. If the two tests each detect all the cases missed by the other, the sensitivity of parallel testing is, of course, 100%. If the two tests are completely independent of each other, then the sensitivity of parallel testing would be 92%.

Parallel testing is particularly useful when the clinician is faced with the need for a very sensitive test but has available only two or more relatively insensitive ones that measure different clinical phenomena. By using the tests in parallel, the net effect is a more sensitive diagnostic strategy. The price, however, is evaluation or treatment of some patients without the disease.

Example PSA and digital rectal exam are both insensitive tests for the diagnosis of prostate cancer (7). Table 3.3 shows their sensitivity, specificity, and predictive values in the screening setting (men without symptoms). When the two tests are used in parallel, the sensitivity increases but the specificity falls. The positive predictive value is lower than for PSA testing alone.

SERIAL TESTING

Physicians most commonly use serial testing strategies in clinical situations where rapid assessment of patients is not required, such as in office practices and hospital clinics in which ambulatory patients are followed over time. Serial testing is also used when some of the tests are expensive or risky, these tests being employed only after simpler and safer tests suggest the presence of disease. For example, maternal age and blood tests (α-fetoprotein, chorionic gonadotropin and estriol) are used to identify pregnancies at higher risk of delivering a baby with Down's syndrome. Mothers found to be at high risk by those tests are then offered amniocentesis (13). Serial testing leads to less laboratory use than parallel testing, because additional evaluation is contingent on prior test results. However, serial testing takes more time because additional tests are ordered only after the results of previous ones become available.

Serial testing maximizes specificity and positive predictive value, but lowers sensitivity and the negative predictive value (see Table 3.3). One ends up surer that positive test results represent disease, but runs an increased risk that disease will be missed. Serial testing is particularly useful when none of the individual tests available to a clinician is highly specific.

If a physician is going to use two tests in series, the process will be

Table 3.3
Tests Characteristics of PSA and Digital Rectal Examination (DRE)[a]

Test	Sensitivity	Specificity	Positive Predictive Value
PSA 4.0 µg/mL	0.67	0.97	0.43
Abnormal DRE	0.50	0.94	0.24
Abnormal PSA or DRE	0.84	0.92	0.28
Abnormal PSA and DRE	0.34	0.995	0.49

[a] PSA and DRE alone and in combination (parallel and serial testing) in the diagnosis of prostate cancer. (Adapted from Kramer BS et al. Prostate cancer screening: what we know and what we need to know. Ann Int Med 1993;119:914–923.)

more efficient if the test with the highest specificity is used first. Table 3.4 shows the effect of sequence on serial testing. Test A is more specific than test B, whereas B is more sensitive than A. By using A first, fewer patients are subjected to both tests, even though equal numbers of diseased patients are diagnosed, regardless of the sequence of tests. However, if one test is much cheaper or less risky, it may be more prudent to use it first.

ASSUMPTION OF INDEPENDENCE

When multiple tests are used, as discussed above, the accuracy of the result depends on whether the additional information contributed by each test is somewhat independent of that already available from the preceding ones, i.e., the next test does not simply duplicate known information. In fact, this premise underlies the entire approach to predictive value we have discussed. However, it seems unlikely that the tests for most diseases

Table 3.4
Effect of Sequence in Serial Testing: A Then B versus B Then A[a]

Prevalence of Disease

| Number of patients tested | 1000 |
| Number of patients with disease | 200 (20% prevalence) |

Sensitivity and Specificity of Tests

Test	Sensitivity	Specificity
A	80	90
B	90	80

Sequence of Testing

Begin with Test A

		Disease +	Disease −	
A	+	160	80	240
	−	40	720	760
		200	800	1000

240 Patients Retested with B

		Disease +	Disease −	
B	+	144	16	160
	−	16	64	80
		160	80	240

Begin with Test B

		Disease +	Disease −	
B	+	180	160	340
	−	20	640	660
		200	800	1000

340 Patients Retested with A

		Disease +	Disease −	
A	+	144	16	160
	−	46	144	180
		180	160	340

[a] Note that in both sequences the same number of patients are identified as diseased (160) and the same number of true positives (144) are identified. But when test A (with the higher specificity) is used first, fewer patients are retested. The lower sensitivity of test A does not adversely affect the final result.

are fully independent of one another. If the assumption that the tests are completely independent is wrong, calculation of the probability of disease from several tests would tend to overestimate the tests' value.

SERIAL LIKELIHOOD RATIOS

When a series of tests is used, an overall probability can be calculated, using the likelihood ratio for each test result, as shown in Figure 3.11. The prevalence of disease before testing is first converted to pretest odds. As each test is done, the posttest odds of one becomes the pretest odds for the next. In the end, a new probability of disease is found that takes into account the information contributed by all the tests in the series.

Responsiveness

The clinical status of patients changes continually either in response to treatment or because of the effects of aging or illness. Clinicians regularly face the question, "Has my patient improved or deteriorated?" The tests used to monitor the clinical course (e.g., symptom severity, functional status) are often somewhat different from those used to diagnose disease, but the assessment of their performance is very similar.

The ability of changes in the value of a test to identify correctly changes in clinical status is called its *responsiveness*. It is conceptually related to the validity of a diagnostic test, except that the presence or absence of a meaningful change in clinical status, not the presence or absence of disease, is the gold standard. The magnitude of a test's responsiveness can be expressed as sensitivity, specificity, and predictive value or as the area under the ROC curve.

> *Example*   Several self-report measures of health and functional status are commonly used to monitor the health of populations and evaluate the effects of treatment. Two such measures are restricted activity days—number of

PRETEST PROBABILITY
↓

Test A   Pretest odds x LR_A = Posttest odds
↓

Test B   Pretest odds x LR_B = Posttest odds
↓

POSTTEST PROBABILITY

Figure 3.11.   Use of likelihood ratios in serial testing.

days on which usual activities were limited by illness or injury—and self-reported health—a question asking respondents to rate their health from excellent to poor compared with others their age. The responsiveness of these measures administered 1 year apart was assessed by comparing changes in each measure between older adults who experienced a major illness during the year and those that did not have a major illness (14). The ROC curves in Figure 3.12 show that the changes in self-reported health performed slightly better than chance in picking up changes in health associated with major illness, while changes in restricted activity days performed much better, accounting for 80% of the area under the ROC curve.

Summary

Diagnostic test performance is judged by comparing the results of the test to the presence of disease in a two-by-two table. All four cells of the table must be filled. When estimating the sensitivity and specificity of a new diagnostic test from information in the medical literature, there must be a gold standard to which the accuracy of the test is compared. The diseased and nondiseased subjects should both resemble the kinds of pa-

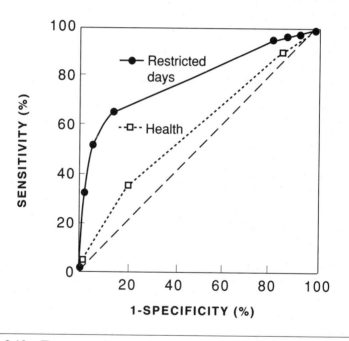

Figure 3.12. The responsiveness of two questionnaire measures of health status. Distinguishing between elderly patients with and without a major intervening illness. (Adapted from Wagner EH, LaCroix AZ, Grothaus LC, Hecht JA. Responsiveness of health status measures to change among older adults. J Am Geriatr Soc 1993;41:241–248.)

tients for whom the test might be useful in practice. In addition, knowledge of the final diagnosis should not bias the interpretation of the test results or vice versa. Changing the cutoff point between normal and abnormal changes sensitivity and specificity. Likelihood ratios are another way of describing the accuracy of a diagnostic test.

The predictive value of a test is the most relevant characteristic when clinicians interpret test results. It is determined not only by sensitivity and specificity of the test but also by the prevalence of the disease, which may change from setting to setting. Usually it is necessary to use several tests, either in parallel or in series, to achieve acceptable diagnostic certainty. Responsiveness, a test's ability to detect change in clinical status, is also judged by the same two-by-two table.

REFERENCES

1. Joint National Committee on Detection, Evaluation, and Treatment of High Blood Pressure. The fifth report of the Joint National Committee on Detection, Evaluation, and Treatment of High Blood Pressure (JNC V). Arch Intern Med 1993;153:154–183.
2. Catalona WJ; et al. Measurement of prostate-specific antigen in serum as a screening test for prostate cancer. N Engl J Med 1991;324:1156–1161.
3. Jensen MC, Brant-Zawadzki MN, Obuchowski N, Modic MT, Malkasian D, Ross JS. Magnetic resonance imaging of the lumbar spine in people without back pain. N Engl J Med 1994;331:69–73.
4. Bartrum RJ Jr, Crow HC, Foote SR. Ultrasonic and radiographic cholecystography. N Engl J Med 1977;296:538–541.
5. Jones TV, Lindsey BA, Yount P, Soltys R, Farani-Enayat B. Alcoholism screening questionnaires: are they vaild in elderly medical outpatients? J Gen Intern Med 1993;8:674–678.
6. Fletcher RH. Carcinoembryonic antigen. Ann Intern Med 1986;104:66–73.
7. Voss JD. Prostate cancer, screening, and prostate-specific antigen: promise or peril? J Gen Intern Med 1994;9:468–474.
8. Barry MJ, Mulley AG, Singer DE. Screening for HTLV III antibodies: the relation between prevalence and positive predictive value and its social consequences. JAMA 1985;253:3395.
9. Ward JW, Grindon AJ, Feorino PM, Schable C, Parvin M, Allen JR. Laboratory and epidemiologic evaluation of an enzyme immunoassay for antibodies to HTLV 111. JAMA 1986;256:357–361.
10. Diamond GA, Forrester JS. Analysis of probability as an aid in the clinical diagnosis of coronary artery disease. N Engl J Med 1979;300:1350–1358.
11. Tierney WM, McDonald CJ. Practice databases and their uses in clinical research. Stat Med 1991;10:541–557.
12. Goldstein BJ, Mushlin AI. Use of a single thyroxine test to evaluate ambulatory medical patients for suspected hypothyroidism. J Gen Intern Med 1987;2:20–24.
13. Haddow JE, Palomaki GE, Knight GJ, Williams J, Pulkkinen A, Canick JA, Saller DN Jr, Bowers GB. Prenatal screening for Down's syndrome with use of maternal serum markers. N Engl J Med 1992;327:588–593.
14. Wagner EH, LaCroix AZ, Grothaus LC, Hecht JA. Responsiveness of health status measures to change among older adults. J Am Geriatr Soc 1993;41:241–248.

SUGGESTED READINGS

Cebul RD, Beck LH. Teaching clinical decision making. New York: Praeger, 1985.
Department of Clinical Epidemiology and Biostatistics, McMaster University. Interpretation of diagnostic data. V. How to do it with simple math. Can Med Assoc J 1983;129:22–29.

(Reprinted in Sackett DL, Haynes RB, Tugwell P, eds. Clinical epidemiology: a basic science for clinical medicine. Boston: Little, Brown, 1985.)

Fagan TJ. Nomogram for Bayes' theorem [Letter]. N Engl J Med 1975;293:257.

Griner PF, Mayewski RJ, Mushlin AI, Greenland P. Selection and interpretation of diagnostic tests and procedures. Principles and applications. Ann Intern Med 1981;94:557–600.

Griner PF, Panzer RJ, Greenland P. Clinical diagnosis and the laboratory: logical strategies for common medical problems. Chicago: Year Book, 1986.

McNeil BJ, Abrams HL, eds, Brigham and Women's Hospital handbook of diagnostic imaging. Boston: Little, Brown, 1986.

Pauker SG, Kassirer JP. Clinical application of decision analysis: a detailed illustration. Semin Nucl Med 1978;8:324–335.

Sheps SB, Schechter MT. The assessment of diagnostic tests. A survey of current medical research. JAMA 1984;252:2418–2422.

Sox HC Jr. Probability theory in the use of diagnostic tests. An introduction to critical study of the literature. Ann Intern Med 1986;104:60–66.

Sox HC Jr, Blatt M, Higgins MC, Marton KI. Medical decision making. Kent, UK: Butterworth, 1987.

Wasson JH, Sox HC Jr, Neff RK, Goldman L. Clinical prediction rules. applications and methodological standards. N Engl J Med 1985;313:793–799.

Weinstein MC, Fineberg HV, Elstein AS, Frazier HS, Neuhauser D, Neutra RR, McNeil BJ. Clinical decision analysis. Philadelphia: WB Saunders, 1980.

4

FREQUENCY

In Chapter 1, we outlined the central questions facing clinicians as they care for patients. In this chapter, we define and describe the quantitative evidence that clinicians use to guide their diagnostic and therapeutic decisions. Let us introduce the subject with a patient.

A 72-year-old man presents with slowly progressive urinary frequency, hesitancy, and dribbling. Digital rectal examination reveals a symmetrically enlarged prostate gland. Urinary flow measurements show significant reduction in flow rate and serum PSA is not elevated. A diagnosis of benign prostatic hyperplasia (BPH) is made. In deciding on treatment, the clinician and patient must weigh the costs and benefits of various therapeutic options: for example, the risks of worsened symptoms or obstructive renal disease with medical treatment versus operative mortality or sexual dysfunction with surgery.

The decisions have traditionally been made by "clinical judgment," which we learn at the bedside and in the clinics. In recent years, methods for quantitative clinical decision making have been introduced into medicine. The most commonly used clinical strategies are decision analysis, cost-effectiveness analysis, and cost-benefit analysis. These methods use quantitative data about the frequency of key clinical events and the consequences of those events to patients to derive the best course of action. The methods, described in more detail at the end of the chapter, are only as good as the estimates of the probability or frequency of clinical outcomes on which they rely.

For the patient with BPH, sound clinical judgment requires accurate information about the probability of symptom deterioration, acute retention or renal damage with medical treatment; and symptom relief, mortality, impotence, or retrograde ejaculation with surgery. These are, in general, the kinds of evidence needed to answer most clinical questions. Decisions are guided by the probability of outcomes under alternative circumstances: in the presence of a positive test versus a negative test or after treatment A versus treatment B. Because the probability of disease, improvement,

75

deterioration, cure, or death forms the basis for answering most clinical questions, this chapter examines measures of clinical frequency.

Assigning Numbers to Probability Statements

Physicians often communicate probabilities as words—*usually, sometimes, rarely*, etc.—rather than as numbers. Substituting words for numbers is convenient and avoids making a precise statement when one is uncertain about a probability. However, it has been shown that there is little agreement about the meanings of commonly used words for frequency.

> *Example* Physicians were asked to estimate the likelihood of disease for each of 30 expressions of probability found by reviewing radiology and laboratory reports. There was great difference of opinion for each expression. Probabilities for *consistent with* ranged from 0.18 to 0.98; for *unlikely*, the range was 0.01–0.93. These data support the authors' assertion that "difference of opinion among physicians regarding the management of a problem may reflect differences in the meaning ascribed to words used to define probability" (1).

Patients also assign widely varying values for expressions of probability. In another study, highly skilled and professional workers thought *usually* referred to probabilities of 0.35–1.0 (±2 standard deviations from the mean); *rarely* meant to them a probability of 0–0.15 (2).

Thus substituting words for numbers diminishes the information conveyed. We advocate using numbers whenever possible.

PERCEPTIONS OF FREQUENCY

Personal experience colors the clinician's perception of the probability of conditions and outcomes. Having a recent patient experience an outcome will tend to make the clinician inflate the probability of that outcome. Conversely, clinicians tend to underestimate the frequency of occurrences that they have not yet experienced or that patients may be reluctant to discuss. For example, systematic interviews of patients after transurethral resection of the prostate gland (TURP) reveal that more than 50% of men experience retrograde ejaculation (3). Most urologists would estimate the frequency to be much lower, since many male patients are reluctant to discuss sexual issues.

Prevalence and Incidence

In general, clinically relevant measures of the frequency or probability of events are fractions in which the numerator is the number of patients experiencing the outcome (cases) and the denominator is the number of people in whom the outcome could have occurred. Such fractions are, of course, proportions; but by common usage, they are referred to as "rates." Clinicians encounter two measures of frequency—prevalence and incidence. A *prevalence* is the fraction (proportion) of a group of people possessing a clinical condition or outcome at a given point in time. Prevalence is measured by surveying a defined population containing people with and without the condition of interest, at a single slice in time. There are two kinds of prevalence. *Point prevalence* is measured at the time of the survey for each person, although not necessarily the same point in time for all the people in the defined population. *Period prevalence* refers to cases that were present at any time during a specific period of time.

An *incidence* is the fraction or proportion of a group initially free of the condition that develops it over a given period of time. Incidence refers then to new cases of disease occurring in a population initially free of the disease or new outcomes, such as disability or death, occurring in patients with a specific disease. As described later in this chapter and in greater detail in Chapter 5, incidence is measured by identifying a susceptible group of people (i.e., people free of the disease or the outcome) and examining them periodically over an interval of time to discover and count new cases that develop during the interval.

> *Example* To illustrate the differences between prevalence and incidence, Figure 4.1 shows the occurrence of disease in a group of 100 people over the course of 3 years (1992–1994). As time passes, individuals in the group develop the disease. They remain in this state until they either recover or die. In the 3 years, 16 people suffer the onset of disease and 4 already had it. The remaining 80 people do not develop disease and do not appear in the figure.
>
> At the beginning of 1992, there are four cases, so the prevalence at that point in time is 4/100. If all 100 individuals, including prior cases, are examined at the beginning of each year, one can compute the prevalence at those points in time. At the beginning of 1993, the prevalence is 5/100 because two of the pre-1992 cases lingered on into 1993 and two of the new cases developing in 1992 terminated (hopefully in a cure) before the examination at the start of 1993. Prevalences can be computed for each of the other two annual examinations, and assuming that none of the original 100 people died, moved away, or refused examination, these prevalences are 7/100 at the beginning of 1994 and 5/100 at the beginning of 1995.
>
> To calculate the incidence of new cases developing in the population, we consider only the 96 individuals free of the disease at the beginning of 1992 and what happens to them over the next 3 years. Five new cases developed in 1992; six new cases developed in 1993, and five additional new cases developed in 1994. The 3-year incidence of the disease is all new cases developing in the 3 years (which is 16) divided by the number of susceptible individuals at the beginning of the follow-up period (96 people), or 16/96 in 3 years. What are the annual incidences for 1992, 1993, and 1994, respectively? Remembering to remove the previous cases from the denominator, we would calculate the annual incidences as 5/96 for 1992, 6/91 for 1993, and 5/85 for 1994.

Every measure of disease frequency necessarily contains some indication of time. With measures of prevalence, time is assumed to be instanta-

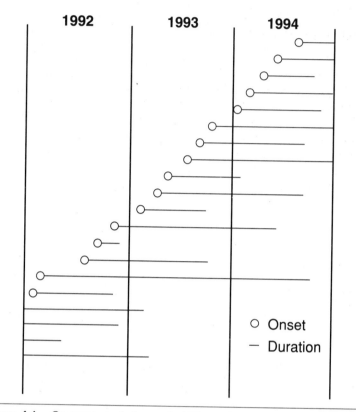

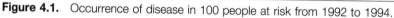

Figure 4.1.   Occurrence of disease in 100 people at risk from 1992 to 1994.

neous, as in a single frame from a motion picture. Prevalence depicts the situation at that point in time for each patient, even though it may, in reality, have taken several weeks or months to collect observations on the various people in the group studied. For incidence, time is the essence because it defines the interval during which susceptible subjects were monitored for the emergence of the event of interest.

Table 4.1 summarizes the characteristics of incidence and prevalence. Although the distinctions between the two seem clear, the literature is replete with misuses of the terms, particularly incidence (4).

Why is it important to know the difference between prevalence and incidence? Because they answer two different questions: (a) What proportion of a group of people have a condition? and (b) At what rate do new cases arise in a group of people as time passes? The answer to one question cannot be obtained directly from the answer to the other.

Measuring Prevalence and Incidence

PREVALENCE STUDIES

The prevalence of disease is measured by surveying a group of people, some of whom are diseased at that point in time while others are healthy (Fig. 4.2). The fraction or proportion of the group that is diseased (i.e., cases) constitutes the prevalence of the disease.

Such one-shot examinations or surveys of a population of individuals, including cases and noncases, are called *prevalence studies*. Another term is *cross-sectional studies*, because people are studied at a point (cross-section) in time. They are among the more common types of research designs reported in the medical literature.

The following is an example of a typical prevalence study.

Table 4.1
Characteristics of Incidence and Prevalence

Characteristic	Incidence	Prevalence
Numerator	New cases occurring during a period of time among a group initially free of disease	All cases counted on a single survey or examination of a group
Denominator	All susceptible people present at the beginning of the period	All people examined, including cases and noncases
Time	Duration of the period	Single point
How measured	Cohort study (see Chapter 5)	Prevalence (cross-sectional) study

Defined Population   **Representative Sample**   **Disease/Outcome Present?**

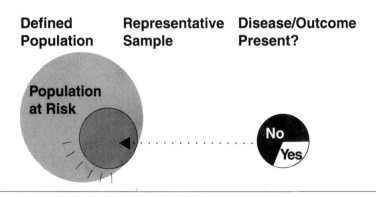

Population at Risk

No   Yes

Figure 4.2. The design of a prevalence survey.

Example   What is the prevalence of dementia in the general population of older adults? To answer this question, 1968 people 75 years of age and older living in Cambridge, England, were surveyed. Each participant underwent an examination that included the Mini-Mental State Examination (MMSE), a test for cognitive impairment. The presence of dementia was identified by a serial testing strategy: Those with MMSE scores of 25 or less were examined using a standardized protocol by a psychiatrist who made the final diagnosis. The prevalence of dementia was about 10% overall, and rates doubled in each 5-year age band (5).

INCIDENCE STUDIES

In contrast to prevalence, incidence is measured by first identifying a population free of the event of interest and then following them through time with periodic examinations to determine occurrences of the event. The population under examination in an incidence study, referred to as a cohort, may be healthy individuals followed for the emergence of disease or diseased individuals followed for outcomes of the disease. This process, also called a cohort study, will be discussed in detail in Chapter 5.

To this point, the term *incidence* has been used to describe the rate of new events in a group of people of fixed size, all of whom are observed over a period of time. This is called *cumulative incidence*, because new cases are accumulated over time.

Example   To study the incidence of dementia, the Cambridge investigators identified a cohort by removing from the follow-up study population those older individuals diagnosed with dementia in the prevalence study described above (6). The remaining 1778 nondemented people were tracked. Of these, 305 died, 190 refused further testing, and 88 could not be found or were too ill to be examined. The remaining 1195 were reexamined an average of 2.5 years after the original examination. Overall, the annual incidence rate of demention in this cohort was 4.3% and exceeded 8% per year for those who were over age 85 at the time of the prevalence examination.

A second approach to estimating incidence is to measure the number of new cases emerging in an ever-changing population, where people are under study and susceptible for varying lengths of time. The incidence measure derived from studies of this type is sometimes called *incidence density*. Typical examples are clinical trials of chronic treatment in which eligible patients are enrolled over several years so that early enrollees are treated and followed longer than late enrollees. In an effort to keep the contribution of individual subjects commensurate with their follow-up interval, the denominator of an incidence density measure is not persons at risk for a specific time period but person-time at risk of the event. An individual followed for 10 years without becoming a case contributes 10 person-years, whereas an individual followed for 1 year contributes only one person-year to the denominator. Incidence density is expressed as the number of new cases per total number of person-years at risk.

The person-years approach is also useful for estimating the incidence of disease in large populations of known size when an accurate count of new cases and an estimate of the population at risk are available, e.g., a population-based cancer registry.

A disadvantage of the incidence density approach is that it lumps together different lengths of follow-up. A small number of patients followed for a long time can contribute as much to the denominator as a large number of patients followed for a short time. If these long-term follow-up patients are systematically different from short-term follow-up patients, the resulting incidence measures may be biased.

Interpreting Measures of Clinical Frequency

To make sense of a prevalence or incidence rate, the first steps involve careful definition of both the numerator and the denominator.

WHAT IS A CASE?—DEFINING THE NUMERATOR

Up to this point, the general term *case* has been used to indicate an individual suffering from the disease or outcome of interest. In classical epidemiology, cases tend to be individuals with a disease, and prevalence and incidence refer to the frequency of cases among population groups like the residents of a community. However, clinical decisions often depend on information about the frequency or rate of disease manifestations, such as symptoms, signs, or laboratory abnormalities, or the frequency of disease outcomes, such as death, disability, or symptomatic improvement. In clinical practice, then, "cases" are often those patients with a disease who manifest a particular clinical finding or experience a particular outcome.

To interpret rates, it is necessary to know the basis on which a case is defined, because the criteria used to define a case can strongly affect rates.

> *Example* One simple way to identify a case is to ask people whether they have a certain condition. How does this method compare to more rigorous methods? In the Commission on Chronic Illness study, the prevalences of various conditions, as determined by personal interviews in the home, were compared with the prevalences as determined by physician examination of the same individuals. Figure 4.3 illustrates the interview prevalences and the clinical examination prevalences for various conditions.
> The data illustrate that these two methods of defining a case can generate very different estimates of prevalence and in different directions, depending on the condition (7).

For some conditions, broadly accepted, explicit diagnostic criteria are available. The Centers for Disease Control and Prevention criteria for definite Lyme disease (Table 4.2) can be used as an example (8). These criteria demonstrate the specificity required to define reliably a disease that is as much in the public eye as is Lyme disease. They also illustrate a trade-off between rigorous definitions and clinical reality. If only "definite" cases

Method of Defining Case

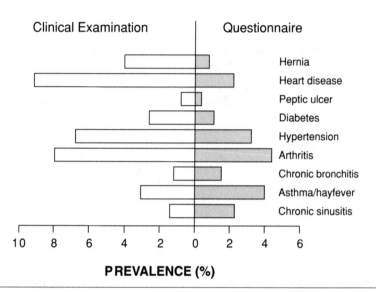

Clinical Examination | Questionnaire

Hernia
Heart disease
Peptic ulcer
Diabetes
Hypertension
Arthritis
Chronic bronchitis
Asthma/hayfever
Chronic sinusitis

10   8   6   4   2   0   2   4   6

PREVALENCE (%)

Figure 4.3.   Prevalence depends on the definition of a case. The prevalence of diseases in the general population based on people's opinions (survey) and clinical evaluation. (Data from Sanders BS. Have morbidity surveys been oversold? Am J Public Health 1962;52:1648–1659.)

Table 4.2
Criteria for Reporting Lyme Disease[a]

Clinical Case Definition (Confirmed)
  Erythema Migrans *or*
  At least one late manifestation *and* laboratory confirmation of infection

Late Manifestation (When Alternative Explanation Not Found)
  Musculoskeletal
    Recurrent brief attacks of objective joint swelling
  Nervous system: any of the following
    Lymphocytic meningitis
    Cranial neuritis (particularly facial palsy)
    Encephalomyelitis with antibody in CSF
  Cardiovascular
    Acute onset 2 or 3° atrioventricular conduction defects that resolve.

Laboratory Confirmation (Any of the Following)
  Isolation of *Borrelia burgdorfei*
  Diagnostic levels of IgM and IgG antibodies to the spirochete in serum or CSF
  Significant change in antibody responses in paired acute- and convalescent-phase serum
    samples.

[a] Centers for Disease Control and Prevention criteria. (Adopted from U.S. Department of Health and Human Services. Case definitions for public health surveillance. MMWR 1990;39:19–20.)

were included in a rate, most patients who ordinarily would be considered to have the disease would not be included. On the other hand, including "probable" cases could overestimate the true rate of disease.

> *Example*   The incidence rate of Lyme disease was estimated in Olmstead County, Minnesota (9). Between 1980 and 1990, 68 cases had been clinically diagnosed in residents of the county. Only 17 (25%) met CDC criteria. In Minnesota, it is mandatory to report Lyme disease to a public health official, yet only 7 cases were reported, of which four met CDC criteria. These data illustrate how difficult it is to make accurate estimates of the frequency of diseases whose diagnosis relies on multiple clinical criteria.

WHAT IS THE POPULATION?—DEFINING THE DENOMINATOR

A rate is useful only to the extent that the individual practitioner can decide to which kinds of patients the rate applies. The size and characteristics of the group of individuals in which the cases arose must be known.

Customarily, the group included in the denominator of a rate is referred to as the population or, more particularly, the *population at risk*, where *at risk* means susceptible to the disease or outcome counted in the numerator. For example, the incidence or prevalence of cervical cancer will be underestimated if the population includes women who have had hysterectomies or includes men.

The denominator of a rate should include the population relevant to the question being asked, or a representative sample of them. But what is relevant depends on one's perspective. For example, if we wanted to know the true prevalence of rheumatoid arthritis in Americans, we would prefer to include in the denominator a random sample of all people in the United States. But if we wanted to know the prevalence of rheumatoid arthritis in medical practice—perhaps to plan services—the relevant denominator would be patients seen in office practice, not people in the population at large. In one survey, only 25% of adults found to have arthritic and rheumatic complaints (not necessarily rheumatoid arthritis) during a community survey had received services for such complaints from any health professional or institution (10).

It is customary for epidemiologists to think of a population as consisting of all individuals residing in a geographic area. And so it should be for studies of cause and effect in the general population. But in studies of clinical questions, the relevant populations generally consist of patients suffering from certain diseases or exhibiting certain clinical findings and who are found in clinical settings that are similar to those in which the information will be used. Commonly, such patients are assembled at a limited number of clinical facilities where academic physicians see patients. They may make up a small and peculiar subset of all patients with the findings in some geographic area and may even be an unusual group for office practice in general.

What difference might the choice of a population make? What is at issue is the generalizability of observed rates.

SAMPLING

It is rarely possible to study all the people who have or might develop the condition of interest. Usually, one takes a sample, so that the number studied is of manageable size. This raises a question: Is the sample representative of the population?

In general, there are two ways to obtain a representative sample. In a *random sample,* every individual in the population has an equal probability of being selected. The more general term *probability sample* is used if every person has a known (not necessarily equal) probability of being selected. It is often important that a study sample includes a sufficient number of members of particular subgroups of interest such as ethnic minorities. If these subgroups are small, a simple random sample of the entire population may not include enough subgroup members. To remedy this, a larger percentage of each of these subgroups is selected at random. The final sample will still be representative of the entire population if the different sampling fractions are accounted for in the analysis. On the average, the characteristics of people in probability samples are similar to those of the population from which they were selected, particularly if a large sample is chosen.

Other methods of selecting samples may well be biased and so do not necessarily represent the parent population. Most groups of patients described in the medical literature, and found in most clinicians' experience, are based on biased samples. Typically, patients are included in studies because they are under care in an academic institution, available, willing to be studied, and perhaps also particularly interesting and/or severely affected. There is nothing wrong with this practice—as long as it is understood to whom the results do (or do not) apply.

Relationship among Incidence, Prevalence, and Duration of Disease

Anything that increases the duration of the disease or clinical finding in a patient will increase the chance that that patient will be identified in a prevalence study. A glance at Figure 4.1 will confirm this. The relationship among incidence and prevalence and duration of disease in a steady state—i.e., where none of the variables is changing much over time—is approximated by the following expression:

$$\text{Prevalence} = \text{Incidence} \times \text{Average duration of the disease}$$

Example   Table 4.3 shows approximate annual incidence and prevalence rates for asthma. Incidence falls with increasing age, illustrating the fact that the disease arises primarily in childhood. But prevalence stays fairly stable over the entire age span, indicating that asthma tends to be chronic and is especially chronic among older individuals. Also, because the pool of prevalent cases does not increase in size, about the same number of patients are recovering from their asthma as new patients are acquiring it.

If we use the following formula, we can determine that asthma has an average duration of 10 years:

$$\text{Average duration} = \text{Prevalence} \div \text{Incidence}$$

When the duration of asthma is determined for each age category by dividing the prevalences by the incidences, it is apparent that the duration of asthma increases with increasing age. This reflects the clinical observation that childhood asthma often clears with time, whereas adult asthma tends to be more chronic.

Bias in Prevalence Studies

Prevalence studies can be used to investigate potentially causal relationships between risk factors and a disease or prognostic factors and an outcome. For this purpose, they are quick but inferior alternatives to incidence studies. Two characteristics of prevalence studies are particularly troublesome: uncertainty about the temporal sequence and biases associated with the study of cases of longer duration—"old" cases.

UNCERTAINTY ABOUT TEMPORAL SEQUENCES

In prevalence studies, disease and the possible factors responsible for the disease are measured simultaneously, and so it is often unclear which came first. The time sequence is obscured, and if it is important to the interpretation it must be inferred. If the risk or prognostic factor is certain to have preceded the onset of disease or outcome—e.g., family history or a genetic marker—interpretation of the cause-and-effect sequence is less worrisome. If the risk or prognostic factor can be a manifestation of the

Table 4.3
The Relationships among Incidence, Prevalence, and Duration of Disease: Asthma in the United States[a]

Age	Annual Incidence	Prevalence	Duration $= \dfrac{\text{Prevalence}}{\text{Annual Incidence}}$
0–5	6/1000	29/1000	4.8 years
6–16	3/1000	32/1000	10.7 years
17–44	2/1000	26/1000	13.0 years
45–64	1/1000	33/1000	33.0 years
65+	0	36/1000	33.0 years
	3/1000	30/1000	10.0 years

[a] Approximated from several sources.

disease or outcome—e.g., an abnormal laboratory test or a psychological state—determining the sequence of events is much more difficult. In contrast, studies of incidence have a built-in sequence of events because possible causes of disease are measured initially, before disease has occurred. These relationships are illustrated in Figure 4.4.

BIASES STUDYING "OLD" CASES

The difference between cases found in the numerator of incidence rates and of prevalences rates is illustrated in Figure 4.5. In an incidence study, all cases are new and most cases occurring in the population at risk can be ascertained if followed carefully through time. In contrast, a prevalence study includes a mixture of old and new cases that are available at the time of the single examination—that is, they identify cases that happen to be both active (i.e., diagnosable) and alive at the time of the survey. Obviously, prevalence rates will be dominated by those patients who are able to survive their disease without losing its manifestations. The differences between the kinds of cases included in the numerator of an incidence and the kinds of cases included in the numerator of a prevalence may influence how the rates are interpreted.

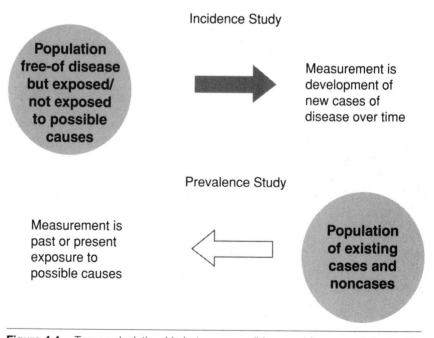

Figure 4.4. Temporal relationship between possible causal factors and disease for incidence and prevalence studies.

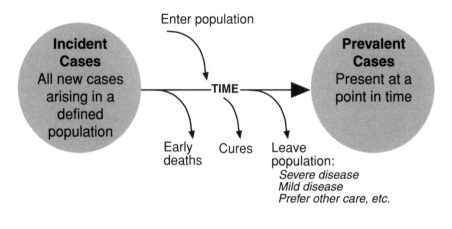

Figure 4.5. The difference in cases for incidence and prevalence studies.

Prevalence is affected by the average duration of disease. Rapidly fatal episodes of a disease would be included in an incidence study, but most would be missed by a prevalence study. For example, 25–40% of all deaths from coronary heart disease occur within 24 hr of the onset of symptoms in people with no prior evidence of disease. A prevalence study would, therefore, underestimate cases of coronary heart disease. On the other hand, diseases of long duration are well represented in prevalence surveys, even if their incidence is low. For example, although the incidence of Crohn's disease is only about 2 to 7 per 100,000/year, its prevalence is more than 100 per 100,000, reflecting the chronic nature of the disease (11).

Prevalence rates also selectively include more severe cases of nonfatal diseases. For example, patients with quiescent rheumatoid arthritis might not be diagnosed in a study based on current symptoms and physical findings. Similarly, patients with recurrent but controllable illnesses, such as congestive heart failure or depression, may be well at a given point in time and, therefore, might not be discovered on a single examination. Unremitting disease, on the other hand, is less likely to be overlooked and, therefore, would contribute disproportionately to the pool of cases assembled by a prevalence study.

Uses of Incidence and Prevalence

What purposes do incidence and prevalence serve? Clinicians use them in three different ways: predicting the future course of a patient, assigning a probability to a patient, and making comparisons.

PREDICTING THE FUTURE

Incidence is a description of the rate at which a disease or a disease outcome has arisen over time in a group of people known to be free of the disease at the beginning of follow-up. It can be used to predict the probability that similar people will develop the condition in the future.

> *Example* The probabilities of outcomes following TURP, needed to decide the most appropriate treatment for the man with BPH described at the opening of this chapter, were estimated from a large cohort study of older men in New England (12). Interviews with more than 300 men undergoing TURP revealed that symptom resolution varied with the severity of symptoms before surgery; 93% of men with severe symptoms improved with surgery while only 79% of those with moderate baseline symptoms improved.

On the other hand, prevalence studies offer no sound basis for predicting the future. If a prevalence study finds that 30% of patients with stroke are depressed, this does not mean that 30% of nondepressed stroke patients will become depressed in the future. It may be that depression predisposes to stroke, that stroke predisposes to depression, or that nondepressed stroke patients recover quickly. To find out the percentage of stroke patients who become depressed, new stroke patients must be followed over time with repeat measures of depressive symptoms.

ASSIGNING A PROBABILITY THAT A PATIENT HAS THE CONDITION

Prevalence studies are particularly useful in guiding decisions about diagnosis and treatment. As pointed out in Chapter 3, knowing that a patient with a combination of demographic and clinical characteristics has a given probability of having a disease influences the use and interpretation of diagnostic tests. It may also may affect the selection among various treatment options.

A patient with pharyngitis illustrates how variations in prevalence or prior probability can influence the approach to a clinical problem.

> *Example* A study compared three approaches to the treatment of pharyngitis. The value of the approaches was judged by weighing the potential benefits of preventing rheumatic fever against the costs of penicillin allergy. The three options were to obtain a throat culture and treat only those patients with throat cultures positive for group A β-hemolytic streptococcus, treat all patients without obtaining a culture, and neither culture nor treat any patient.
>
> The analysis revealed that the optimal strategy depended on the likelihood that a patient would have a positive culture, which can be estimated from the prevalence of streptococcal infection in the community at the time and the presence or absence of fever. The authors concluded that if the probability of a positive culture for an individual patient exceeds 20%, the patient should be treated; if it is less than 5%, the patient should not be cultured or treated; and if the probability lies between 5 and 20%, the patient should be cultured first and treated based on the result (13).

This study represents a rational approach to the use of prevalences as indicators of individual probabilities of disease in guiding clinical decision making.

MAKING COMPARISONS

Although isolated incidences and prevalences are useful descriptions, they become much more powerful tools in support of decision making when used to make comparisons. It is the comparison between the frequencies of disease among individuals with certain characteristics and individuals not sharing those characteristics that provides the strongest evidence. For example, the risk (incidence) of lung cancer among males who smoke heavily is of the order of 0.17% per year, hardly a common event. Only when this incidence is contrasted with the incidence in nonsmokers (approximately 0.007% per year) does the devastating effect of smoking emerge. Clinicians use measures of frequency as the ingredients in comparative measures of the association between a factor and the disease or disease outcome. Ways of comparing rates are described in more detail in Chapter 5.

Clinical Decision Analysis

Quantitative approaches to assisting in decision making have been used to define the most effective and efficient way to deal with specific problems in individual patients (*clinical policy*) or for allocating resources to larger groups of people, such as communities or political jurisdictions (*public policy*).

In *decision analysis,* one sets out alternative courses of action (e.g., surgery versus medical treatment for BPH or culture then treat or treat everybody for streptococcal pharyngitis) and then calculates which choice is likely to result in the most valued outcome, based on estimates of frequencies for each branch in the sequences of events and judgments about the relative value of the possible outcomes. The basic steps are clearly presented elsewhere (14) and are described only briefly below.

1. *Create a decision tree.* Clinical decision analysis begins with a patient who poses a dilemma. Which of the possible courses of action should be taken? The tree begins with these alternative decisions, then branches out to include all of the important consequences of those decisions, and ends with the clinically important outcomes. Branch points involve either patient care decisions ("choice nodes," indicated by squares) or spontaneous events ("chance nodes," indicated by circles). Although there is an infinite number of sequences of events and outcomes, usually only a small number are truly important and are reasonably likely to occur. To make the analysis manageable, it is necessary to "prune" the tree so that only the most important branches are included—typically no more than several branch points.

2. *Assign probabilities to chance nodes.* These probabilities are assessments of the frequency of clinical events, which are usually derived from the medical literature.
3. *Assign utilities to the outcomes.* Utilities are quantitative expressions of the relative value of the various outcomes considered. They are best obtained from patients who may confront the decision. The units are arbitrary, but must be on an interval scale, e.g., 0 to 100. It may seem awkward to put a number on the respective values of the various outcomes (death, suffering, loss of function), especially when they are measured in different units, such as the length and quality of life. But patients attach values to outcomes in any case, and the numbers only make the values explicit.
4. *Calculate the expected utilities* for the alternative courses of action. Starting with utilities (at the end of the branches, to the right), multiply utilities by probabilities for each branch and add branches at each node in succession until the expected utility at the main branch point, the decision that has to be made, is reached.
5. *Select the choice* with the highest expected utility.
6. *Sensitivity analysis.* Estimates of probabilities and utilities are uncertain in the first place. The final step in decision analysis is to see how the results of the analysis change as these estimates are varied over a range of plausible values. That is, one must find out how "sensitive" the decision is to imprecision in the estimates. Sensitivity analysis indicates which point in the sequence of events have the most effect on the decision and how large the effect might be.

> ***Example***   The therapeutic options facing the older man with urinary symptoms from benign prostatic hyperplasia (described at the opening of this chapter) have been evaluated using decision analysis (15). Before drugs and laser prostatectomy made the decision more complicated, the options were surgery (transurethral resection of the prostate, TURP) or careful follow-up, called "watchful waiting." Figure 4.6 shows the decision tree that the authors used to evaluate the options. The frequencies of the various outcomes were derived in the incidence study of New England men described earlier in the chapter (12) and other published sources (15). Note that the optimal decision in this case is surgery (net utility 0.94). In this case, TURP is the favored treatment because the risk of operative death is low and the utilities assigned to incontinence or impotence are the same as that assigned to living with stable moderate urinary symptoms. If stable moderate symptoms were preferred over incontinence or impotence, the balance would shift.

Summary

Most clinical questions are answered by reference to the frequency of events under varying circumstances. The frequency of clinical events is indicated by probabilities or fractions, the numerators of which include

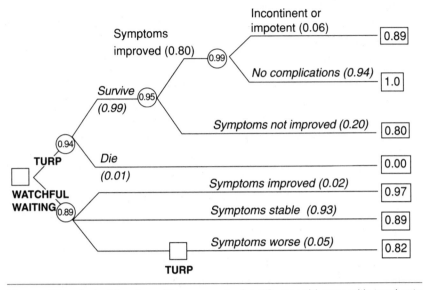

Figure 4.6. A decision tree. Management of a 70-year-old man with moderate symptoms from benign prostatic hyperplasia. (Data adapted from Barry MJ, Mulley AG, Fowler FJ, Wennberg JW. Watchful waiting vs. immediate transurethral resection for symptomatic prostatism. JAMA 1988; 259(20):3010–3017.)

the number of cases and the denominators of which include the number of people from whom the cases arose.

There are two measures of frequency: prevalence and incidence. Prevalence is the proportion of a group with the disease at a single point in time. Incidence is the proportion of a susceptible group that develops new cases of the disease over an interval of time.

Prevalence is measured by a single survey of a group containing cases and noncases, whereas measurement of incidence requires examinations of a previously disease-free group over time. Thus prevalence studies identify only those cases who are alive and diagnosable at the time of the survey, whereas cohort (incidence) studies ascertain all new cases. Prevalent cases, therefore, may be a biased subset of all cases because they do not include those who have already succumbed or been cured. In addition, prevalence studies frequently do not permit a clear understanding of the temporal relationship between a causal factor and a disease.

To make sense of incidence and prevalence, the clinician must understand the basis on which the disease is diagnosed and the characteristics of the population represented in the denominator. The latter is of particular importance in trying to decide if a given measure of incidence or prevalence pertains to patients in one's own practice.

Incidence is the most appropriate measure of frequency with which to predict the future. Prevalence serves to quantitate the likelihood that a patient with certain characteristics has the disease at a single point in time and is used for decisions about diagnosis and screening. The most powerful use of incidence and prevalence, however, is to compare different clinical alternatives.

Measures of disease or outcome incidence are essential ingredients in methods for quantitative decision making. Approaches such as decision analysis define alternative clinical strategies and then evaluate those strategies quantitatively by comparing their expected utilities determined from the frequencies and values assigned to the major outcomes associated with each strategy.

Postscript

Counting clinical events as described in this chapter may seem to be the most mundane of tasks. It seems so obvious that examining counts of clinical events under various circumstances is the foundation of clinical science. It may be worth reminding the reader that Pierre Louis introduced the "numerical method" of evaluating therapy less than 200 years ago. Louis had the audacity to count deaths and recoveries from febrile illness in the presence and absence of blood-letting. He was vilified for allowing lifeless numbers to cast doubt on the healing powers of the leech, powers that had been amply confirmed by decades of astute qualitative clinical observation.

REFERENCES

1. Bryant GD, Norman GR. Expressions of probability: words and numbers. N Engl J Med 1980;302:411.
2. Toogood JH. What do we mean by "usually"? Lancet 1980;1:1094.
3. McConnell JD, Barry MJ, Bruskewitz RC. Benign prostatic hyperplasia: diagnosis and treatment. Clin Pract Guide Quick Ref Guide Clin 1994;8:1–17.
4. Friedman GD. Medical usage and abusage, "prevalence" and "incidence." Ann Intern Med 1976;84:502–503.
5. O'Connor DW, Politt PA, Hyde JB, Fellows JL, Miller ND, Brook CPB, Reiss BB, Roth M. The prevalence of dementia as measured by the Cambridge Mental Disorders of the Elderly Examiniation. Acta Psychiatr Scand 1989;79:190–198.
6. Paykel ES, Brayne C, Huppert FA, Gill C, Barkley C, Gehlhaar E, Beardsall L, Girling DM, Pollitt P, O'Connor D. Incidence of dementia in a population older that 75 years in the United Kingdom. Arch Gen Psychiatry 1994;51:325–332.
7. Sanders BS. Have morbidity surveys been oversold? Am J Public Health 1962;52:1648–1659.
8. Case definitions for public health surveillance. MMRW 1990;(RR-13):19–21.
9. Matteson EL, Beckett VL, O'Fallon WM, Melton LJ III, Duffy J. Epidemiology of Lyme disease in Olmsted County, MN, 1975–1990. J Rheumatol 1992;19:1743–1745.
10. Spitzer WO, Harth M, Goldsmith CH, Norman GR, Dickie GL, Bass MJ, Newell JP. The arthritic complaint in primary care: prevalence, related disability, and costs. J Rheumatol 1976;3:88–99.

11. Sedlack RE, Whisnant J, Elveback LR, Kurland LT. Incidence of Crohn's disease in Olmstec County, Minnesota, 1935–1975. Am J Epidemiol 1980;112:759–763.

12. Fowler FJ, Wennberg JE, Timothy RP, Barry MJ, Mulley AG, Hanley D. Symptom status and quality of life following prostatectomy. JAMA 1988;259:3018–3022.

13. Tompkins RK, Burnes DC, Cable WE. An analysis of the cost-effectiveness of pharyngitis management and acute rheumatic fever prevention. Ann Intern Med 1977;86:481–492.

14. Sox HC, Blatt MA, Higgins MC, Marton KI. Medical decision making. Stoneham, MA: Butterworth, 1988.

15. Barry MJ, Mulley AG, Fowler FJ, Wennberg JW. Watchful waiting vs. immediate transurethral resection for symptomatic prostatism. JAMA 1988;259:3010–3017.

SUGGESTED READINGS

Ellenberg JH, Nelson KB. Sample selection and the natural history of disease: studies of febrile seizures. JAMA 1980;243(1):377–1340.

Friedman GD. Medical usage and abusage, "prevalence" and "incidence." Ann Intern Med 1976;84:502–503.

Morgenstern H, Kleinbaum DG, Kupper LL. Measures of disease incidence used in epidemiologic research. Int J Epidemiol 1980;9:97–104.

5

RISK

Risk generally refers to the probability of some untoward event. In this chapter, the term *risk* is used in a more restricted sense to indicate the likelihood that people who are exposed to certain factors ("risk factors") will subsequently develop a particular disease.

People have a strong interest in their risk of disease. This concern has spawned many popular books about risk reduction and is reflected in newspaper headlines about the risk of breast cancer from exposure to toxic chemicals, of AIDS from blood transfusions, or of prostatic cancer after vasectomy.

This chapter describes how investigators obtain estimates of risk by observing the relationship between exposure to possible risk factors and the subsequent incidence of disease. We discuss several ways of comparing risks, as they affect both individuals and populations.

Risk Factors

Characteristics that are associated with an increased risk of becoming diseased are called *risk factors*. Some risk factors are inherited. For example, having the haplotype HLA-B27 greatly increases one's risk of acquiring the spondylarthropathies. Work on the Human Genome Project has identified several other diseases for which specific genes are risk factors, including colon cancer, osteoporosis, and amyotropic lateral sclerosis. Other risk factors, such as infectious agents, drugs, and toxins, are found in the physical environment. Still others are part of the social environment. For example, bereavement due to the loss of a spouse, change in daily routines, and crowding all have been shown to increase rates of disease—not only emotional illness but physical illness as well. Some of the most powerful risk factors are behavioral; examples are smoking, drinking alcohol to excess, driving without seat belts, and engaging in unsafe sex.

Exposure to a risk factor means that a person has, before becoming ill, come in contact with or has manifested the factor in question. Exposure can take place at a single point in time, as when a community is exposed

94

to radiation during a nuclear accident. More often, however, contact with risk factors for chronic disease takes place over a period of time. Cigarette smoking, hypertension, sexual promiscuity, and sun exposure are examples.

There are several different ways of characterizing the amount of exposure or contact with a putative risk factor: ever exposed, current dose, largest dose taken, total cumulative dose, years of exposure, years since first contact, etc. (1). Although the various measures of dose tend to be related to each other, some may show an exposure-disease relationship, whereas others do not. For example, cumulative doses of sun exposure constitute a risk factor for nonmelanoma skin cancer, whereas episodes of severe sunburn are a better predictor of melanoma. Choice of an appropriate measure of exposure to a risk factor is usually based on all that is known about the biologic effects of the exposure and the pathophysiology of the disease.

Recognizing Risk

Large risks associated with effects that occur rapidly after exposure are easy for anyone to recognize. Thus it is not difficult to appreciate the relationship between exposure and disease for conditions such as chickenpox, sunburn, and aspirin overdose, because these conditions follow exposure relatively rapidly and with obvious effects. But most morbidity and mortality is caused by chronic diseases. For these, relationships between exposure and disease are far less obvious. It becomes virtually impossible for individual clinicians, however astute, to develop estimates of risk based on their own experiences with patients. This is true for several reasons, which are discussed below.

LONG LATENCY

Many diseases have long latency periods between exposure to risk factors and the first manifestations of disease. This is particularly true for certain cancers, such as thyroid cancer in adults after radiation treatment for childhood tonsillitis. When patients experience the consequence of exposure to a risk factor years later, the original exposure may be all but forgotten. The link between exposure and disease is thereby obscured.

FREQUENT EXPOSURE TO RISK FACTORS

Many risk factors, such as cigarette smoking or eating a diet high in cholesterol and saturated fats, are so common in our society that for many years they scarcely seemed dangerous. Only by comparing patterns of disease among people with and without these risk factors or by investigating special subgroups—e.g., Mormons (who do not smoke) and vegetarians (who eat diets low in cholesterol)—did we recognize risks that are, in fact, large.

LOW INCIDENCE OF DISEASE

Most diseases, even ones thought to be "common," are actually quite rare. Thus, although lung cancer is the most common cause of cancer deaths in Americans, the yearly incidence of lung cancer even in heavy smokers is less than 2 in 1000. In the average physician's practice, years may pass between patients with new cases of lung cancer. It is difficult to draw conclusions about such infrequent events.

SMALL RISK

If a factor confers only a small risk for a disease, a large number of people are required to observe a difference in disease rates between exposed and unexposed persons. This is so even if both the risk factor and the disease occur relatively frequently. For example, it is still uncertain whether birth control pills increase the risk of breast cancer, because estimates of this risk are all small and, therefore, easily discounted as resulting from bias or chance. In contrast, it is not controversial that hepatitis B infection is a risk factor for hepatoma, because people with hepatitis B infection are hundreds of times more likely to get liver cancer than those without it.

COMMON DISEASE

If a disease is common—heart disease, cancer, or stroke—and some of the risk factors for it are already known, it becomes difficult to distinguish a new risk factor from the others. Also, there is less incentive to look for new risk factors. For example, the syndrome of sudden, unexpected death in adults is a common way to die. Many cases seem related to coronary heart disease. However, it is entirely conceivable that there are other important causes, as yet unrecognized because an adequate explanation for most cases is available.

On the other hand, rare diseases and unusual clinical presentations invite efforts to find a cause. AIDS was such an unusual syndrome that the appearance of just a few cases raised suspicion that some new agent (as it turned out, a retrovirus) might be responsible. Similarly, physicians were quick to notice when several cases of carcinoma of the vagina, a very rare condition, began appearing. A careful search for an explanation was undertaken, and maternal exposure to diethylstilbestrol was found.

MULTIPLE CAUSES AND EFFECTS

There is usually not a close, one-to-one relationship between a risk factor and a particular disease. The relationship between hypertension and congestive failure is an example (Fig. 5.1). Some people with hypertension

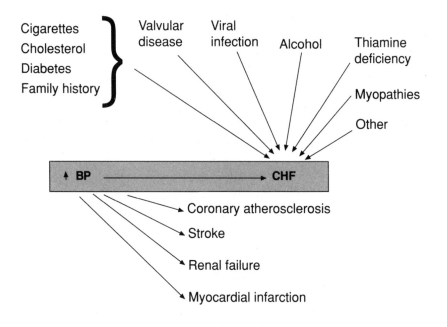

Figure 5.1. Relationship between risk factors and disease: hypertension (↑ BP) and congestive heart failure (CHF). Hypertension causes many diseases, including congestive heart failure, and congestive heart failure has many causes, including hypertension.

develop congestive heart failure and many do not. Also, many people who do not have hypertension develop congestive heart failure, because there are several different causes. The relationship is also obscured because hypertension causes several diseases other than congestive heart failure. Thus, although people with hypertension are about 3 times more likely than those without hypertension to develop congestive heart failure and hypertension is the leading cause of the condition, physicians were not particularly attuned to this relationship until the 1970s, when adequate data became available after careful study of large numbers of people over many years.

For all these reasons, individual clinicians are rarely in a position to confirm associations between exposure and disease, though they may suspect them. For accurate information, they must turn to the medical literature, particularly to studies that are carefully constructed and involve a large number of patients.

Uses of Risk

PREDICTION

Risk factors are used, first and foremost, to predict the occurrence of disease. In fact, risk factors, by definition, predict some future event. The best available information for predicting disease in an individual person is past experience with a large number of people with a similar risk factor. The quality of such predictions depends on the similarity of the people on whom the estimate is based and the person for whom the prediction is made.

It is important to keep in mind that the presence of even a strong risk factor does not mean that an individual is very likely to get the disease. For example, studies have shown that a heavy smoker has a 20-fold greater risk of lung cancer compared with nonsmokers, but he or she still has only a 1 in a 100 chance of getting lung cancer in the next 10 years.

There is a basic incompatibility between the incidence of a disease in groups of people and the chance that an individual will contract that disease. Quite naturally, both patients and clinicians would like to answer questions about the future occurrence of disease as precisely as possible. They are uncomfortable about assigning a probability, such as the chances that a person will get lung cancer or stroke in the next 5 years. Moreover, any one person will, at the end of 5 years, either have the disease or not. So in a sense, the average is always wrong because the two are expressed in different terms, a probability versus the presence or absence of disease. Nevertheless, probabilities can guide clinical decision making. Even if a prediction does not come true in an individual patient, it will usually be borne out in many such patients.

CAUSE

Just because risk factors predict disease, it does not necessarily follow that they cause disease. A risk factor may mark a disease outcome indirectly, by virtue of an association with some other determinant(s) of disease, i.e., it may be confounded with a causal factor. For example, lack of maternal education is a risk factor for low birth weight infants. Yet, other factors related to education, such as poor nutrition, less prenatal care, cigarette smoking, etc., are more directly the causes of low birth weight.

A risk factor that is not a cause of disease is called a *marker*, because it "marks" the increased probability of disease. Not being a cause does not diminish the value of a risk factor as a way of predicting the probability of disease, but it does imply that removing the risk factor might not remove the excess risk associated with it. For example, as pointed out in Chapter 1, although there is growing evidence that the human papillomavirus (HPV) is a risk factor for cervical cancer, the role of other sexually transmitted diseases, such as herpes simplex virus and *Chlamydia*, is not as clear. Antibodies to these agents are more common among patients with cervical cancer than in women without cancer, but the agents may be markers for risk of cervical cancer rather than causes. If so, curing them would not necessarily prevent cervical cancer. On the other hand, decreasing promiscuity might prevent the acquisition of both the causative agent for cervical cancer and other sexually transmitted diseases (2).

There are several ways of deciding whether a risk factor is a cause or merely a marker for disease. These are covered in Chapter 11.

DIAGNOSIS

Knowledge of risk can be used in the diagnostic process, since the presence of a risk factor increases the prevalence (probability) of disease among patients—one way of improving the positive predictive value of a diagnostic test.

However, in individual patients, risk factors usually are not as strong predictors of disease as are clinical findings of early disease. As Rose (3) put it:

> Often the best predictor of future major diseases is the presence of existing minor disease. A low ventilatory function today is the best predictor of its future rate of decline. A high blood pressure today is the best predictor of its future rate of rise. Early coronary heart disease is better than all of the conventional risk factors as a predictor of future fatal disease.

Risk factors can provide the most help with diagnosis in situations where the factor confers a substantial risk and the prevalence of the disease is increased by clinical findings. For example, age and sex are relatively strong risk factors for coronary artery disease, yet the prevalence of disease in the most at risk age and sex group, old men, is only 12%. When specifics of the clinical situation, such as presence and type of chest pain and results of an electrocardiographic stress test, are considered as well, the prevalence of coronary disease can be raised to 99% (4).

More often, it is helpful to use the absence of a risk factor to help rule out disease, particularly when one factor is strong and predominant. Thus it is reasonable to consider mesothelioma in the differential diagnosis of a pleural mass in a patient who is an asbestos worker, but mesothelioma is a much less likely diagnosis for the patient who has never worked with asbestos.

Knowledge of risk factors is also used to improve the efficiency of screening programs by selecting subgroups of patients at increased risk.

PREVENTION

If a risk factor is also a cause of disease, its removal can be used to prevent disease whether or not the mechanism by which the disease takes place is known. Some of the classic successes in the history of epidemiology illustrate this point. For example, before bacteria were identified, Snow found an increased rate of cholera among people drinking water supplied by a particular company and controlled an epidemic by cutting off that supply. More recently, even before HIV had been identified, studies showed that a lifestyle of multiple sexual partners among homosexual men was a risk factor for acquiring AIDS (5). The concept of cause and its relationship to prevention is discussed in Chapter 11.

Studies of Risk

The most powerful way of determining whether exposure to a potential risk factor results in an increased risk of disease is to conduct an experiment. People currently without disease would be divided into groups of equal susceptibility to the disease in question. One group would be exposed to the purported risk factor and the other would not, but the groups would otherwise be treated the same. Later, any difference in observed rates of disease in the groups could be attributed to the risk factor.

Unfortunately, the effects of most risk factors for humans cannot be studied with *experimental studies,* in which the researcher determines who is exposed. Consider some of the questions of risk that concern us today. How much are inactive people at increased risk for cardiovascular disease, everything else being equal? Do cellular phones cause brain cancer? Does alcohol increase the risk of breast cancer? For such questions as these, it is usually not possible to conduct an experiment. First, the experiment would have to go on for decades. Second, it would be unethical to impose possible risk factors on a group of the people in the study. Finally, most people would balk at having their diets and behaviors determined by others for long periods of time. As a result, it is usually necessary to study risk in less obtrusive ways.

Clinical studies in which the researcher gathers data by simply observing events as they happen, without playing an active part in what takes place, are called *observational studies.* Most studies of risk are observational studies, either *cohort studies,* described in the rest of this chapter, or *case control studies,* described in Chapter 10.

COHORTS

The term *cohort* is used to describe a group of people who have something in common when they are first assembled and who are then observed for a period of time to see what happens to them. Table 5.1 lists some of the ways in which cohorts are used in clinical research. Whatever members of a cohort have in common, observations of them should fulfill two criteria if they are to provide sound information about risk.

First, cohorts should be observed over a meaningful period of time in the natural history of the disease in question. This is so there will be

Table 5.1
Cohorts and Their purposes

Characteristic in Common	To Assess Effect of	Example
Age	Age	Life expectancy for people age 70 (regardless of when born)
Date of birth	Calendar time	Tuberculosis rates for people born in 1910
Exposure	Risk factor	Lung cancer in people who smoke
Disease	Prognosis	Survival rate for patients with breast cancer
Preventive intervention	Prevention	Reduction in incidence of pneumonia after pneumococcal vaccination
Therapeutic intervention	Treatment	Improvement in survival for patients with Hodgkin's disease given combination chemotherapy

sufficient time for the risk to be expressed. If we wish to learn whether neck irradiation during childhood results in thyroid neoplasms, a 5-year follow-up would not be a fair test of the hypothesis that thyroid cancer is associated with irradiation, because the usual time period between irradiation exposure and the onset of disease is considerably longer.

Second, all members of the cohort should be observed over the full period of follow-up. To the extent that people drop out of the study and their reasons for dropping out are related in some way to the outcome, the information provided by an incomplete cohort can be a distortion of the true state of affairs.

COHORT STUDIES

In a *cohort study* (Fig. 5.2), a group of people (a cohort) is assembled, none of whom has experienced the outcome of interest, but all of whom could experience it. (For example, in a study of risk factors for endometrial cancer, each member of the cohort should have an intact uterus.) On entry to the study, people in the cohort are classified according to those characteristics (possible risk factors) that might be related to outcome. These people are then observed over time to see which of them experience the outcome. It is then possible to see how initial characteristics relate to subsequent outcome events. Other names for cohort studies are *longitudinal* (emphasizing that patients are followed over time), *prospective* (implying the forward direction in which the patients are pursued), and *incidence* (calling attention to the basic measure of new disease events over time).

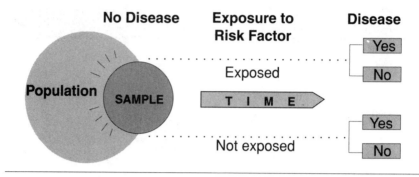

Figure 5.2.   Design of a cohort study of risk.

The following is a description of a classical cohort study, which has made important contributions to our understanding of cardiovascular disease.

> *Example*   The Framingham Study (6) was begun in 1949 to identify factors associated with an increased risk of coronary heart disease (CHD). A representative sample of 5,209 men and women, aged 30–59, was selected from approximately 10,000 persons of that age living in Framingham, a small town near Boston. Of these, 5,127 were free of CHD when first examined and, therefore, were at risk of developing CHD. These people were reexamined biennially for evidence of coronary disease. The study ran for 30 years and demonstrated that risk of developing CHD is associated with elevated blood pressure, high serum cholesterol, cigarette smoking, glucose intolerance, and left ventricular hypertrophy. There was a large difference in risk between those with none and those with all of these risk factors.

HISTORICAL COHORT STUDIES

Cohort studies can be conducted in two ways (Fig. 5.3). The cohort can be assembled in the present and followed into the future (a *concurrent cohort study*), or it can be identified from past records and followed forward from that time up to the present (an *historical cohort study*).

Most of the advantages and disadvantages of cohort studies discussed below apply whether the study is concurrent or historical. However, the potential for difficulties with the quality of data is different for the two. In concurrent studies, data can be collected specifically for the purposes of the study and with full anticipation of what is needed. It is thereby possible to avoid biases that might undermine the accuracy of the data. On the other hand, data for historical cohorts are often gathered for other purposes—usually as part of medical records for patient care. These data may not be of sufficient quality for rigorous research.

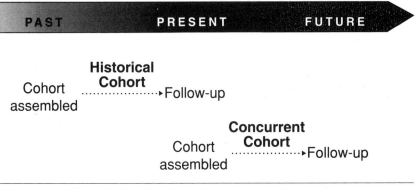

PAST   PRESENT   FUTURE

Historical
Cohort   **Cohort** ·················▸Follow-up
assembled

                         Concurrent
                Cohort   **Cohort** ··············▸Follow-up
                assembled

Figure 5.3. Historical and concurrent cohort studies.

ADVANTAGES AND DISADVANTAGES OF COHORT STUDIES

Some of the advantages and disadvantages of cohort studies, for the purpose of describing risk factors, are summarized in Table 5.2. Cohort studies of risk are the best available substitutes for a true experiment when experimentation is not possible. They follow the same logic as a clinical trial, and they allow determination of exposure to a possible risk factor while avoiding any possibility of bias that might occur if exposure is determined after the outcome is already known.

The principal disadvantage is that if the outcome is infrequent (which is usually the case) a large number of people must be entered in a study and remain under observation for a long time before results are available. For example, the Framingham Study of coronary heart disease—one of the most frequent of the chronic diseases in America—was the largest

Table 5.2
Advantages and Disadvantages of Cohort Studies

Advantages	Disadvantages
The only way of establishing incidence (i.e., absolute risk) directly	Inefficient because many more subjects must be enrolled than experience the event of interest; therefore, cannot be used for rare diseases
Follows the same logic as the clinical question: If persons exposed, then do they get the disease?	Expensive because of resources necessary to study many people over time
Exposure can be elicited without the bias that might occur if outcome were already known	Results not available for a long time
Can assess the relationship between exposure and many diseases	Assesses the relationship between disease and exposure to only relatively few factors (i.e., those recorded at the outset of the study)

study of its kind when it began. Nevertheless, more than 5000 people had to be followed for several years before the first, preliminary conclusions could be published. Only 5% of the people had experienced a coronary event during the first 8 years!

A related problem with cohort studies results from the fact that the people being studied are usually "free living" and not under the control of researchers. A great deal of effort and money must be expended to keep track of them. Cohort studies, therefore, are expensive, sometimes costing many millions of dollars.

Because of the time and money required for cohort studies, this approach cannot be used for all clinical questions about risk. For practical reasons, the cohort approach has been reserved for only the most important questions. This has led to efforts to find more efficient, yet dependable, ways of assessing risk. (The most common of these, case control studies, is discussed in Chapter 10.)

The most important scientific disadvantage of observational studies, including cohort studies, is that they are subject to a great many more potential biases than are experiments. People who are exposed to a certain risk factor in the natural course of events are likely to differ in a great many ways from a comparison group of people not exposed to the factor. If these other differences are also related to the disease in question, they could account for any association observed between the putative risk factor and the disease.

This leads to the main challenge of observational studies: to deal with extraneous differences between exposed and nonexposed groups to mimic as closely as possible an experiment. The differences are considered "extraneous" from the point of view of someone trying to determine cause-and-effect relationships. The following example illustrates one approach to handling such differences.

> *Example* Although the presence of sickle-cell trait (HbAS) is generally regarded as a benign condition, several studies have suggested that it is associated with defects in physical growth and cognitive development. A study was undertaken, therefore, to see if children born with HbAS experienced problems in growth and development more frequently than children with normal hemoglobin (HbAA), everything else being equal (7). It was recognized that a great many other factors are related to growth and development and also to having HbAS. Among these are race, sex, birth date, birth weight, gestational age, 5-min Apgar score, and socioeconomic status. If these other factors were not taken into account, one or more of them could bias the results of the study, and it would not be possible to distinguish the effects of HbAS, in and of itself, from the effects of the other factors. The authors chose to deal with these other factors by matching. For each child with HbAS, they selected a child with HbAA who was similar with respect to the seven other factors. A total of 100 newborns—50 with HbAS and 50 with HbAA—

were followed from birth to 3–5 years old. No differences in growth and development were found.

Major biases in observational studies and ways of dealing them are described in Chapter 6.

Comparing Risks

The basic expression of risk is incidence, defined in Chapter 4 as the number of new cases of disease arising in a defined population during a given period of time. But usually we want to compare the incidence of disease in two or more groups in a cohort that differ in exposure to a possible risk factor. To compare risks, several measures of the association between exposure and disease, called *measures of effect,* are commonly used. They represent different concepts of risk and are used for different purposes. Four measures of effect are discussed below (Tables 5.3 and 5.4).

ATTRIBUTABLE RISK

First, one might ask, "What is the additional risk (incidence) of disease following exposure, over and above that experienced by people who are not exposed?" The answer is expressed as *attributable risk,* the incidence of disease in exposed persons minus the incidence in nonexposed persons. Attributable risk is the additional incidence of disease related to exposure, taking into account the background incidence of disease, presumably from other causes. Note that this way of comparing rates implies that the risk factor is a cause and not just a marker. Because of the way it is calculated, attributable risk is also called *risk difference.*

Table 5.3
Measures of Effect

Expression	Question	Definition[a]
Attributable risk (risk difference)	What is the incidence of disease attributable to exposure?	$AR = I_E - I_{\overline{E}}$
Relative risk (risk ratio)	How many times more likely are exposed persons to become diseased, relative to nonexposed persons?	$RR = \dfrac{I_E}{I_{\overline{E}}}$
Population attributable risk	What is the incidence of disease in a population, associated with the occurrence of a risk factor?	$AR_P = AR \times P$
Population attributable fraction	What fraction of disease in a population is attributable to exposure to a risk factor?	$AF_P = \dfrac{AR_P}{I_T}$

[a] Where I_E = incidence in exposed persons; $I_{\overline{E}}$ = incidence in nonexposed persons; P = prevalence of exposure to a risk factor; and I_T = total incidence of disease in a population.

Table 5.4
Calculating Measures of Effect: Cigarette Smoking and Death from Lung Cancer[a]

Simple risks	
Death rate from lung cancer in cigarette smokers	0.96/1000/year
Death rate from lung cancer in nonsmokers	0.07/1000/year
Prevalence of cigarette smoking	56%
Total death rate from lung cancer	0.56/1000/year

Compared risks

Attributable risk = 0.96/1000/year − 0.07/1000/year
        = 0.89/1000/year
Relative risk = 0.96/1000/year ÷ 0.07/1000/year
        = 13.7
Population attributable risk = 0.89/1000/year × 0.56
        = 0.50/1000/year
Population attributable fraction = 0.50/1000/year ÷ 0.56/1000/year
        = 0.89

[a] Estimated data from Doll R, Hill AB. Br Med J 1964;1:1399–1410.

RELATIVE RISK

On the other hand, one might ask, "How many times are exposed persons more likely to get the disease relative to nonexposed persons?" To answer this question, we speak of *relative risk* or *risk ratio*, the ratio of incidence in exposed persons to incidence in nonexposed persons. Relative risk tells us nothing about the magnitude of absolute risk (incidence). Even for large relative risks, the absolute risk might be quite small if the disease is uncommon. It does tell us the strength of the association between exposure and disease and so is a useful measure of effect for studies of disease etiology.

INTERPRETING ESTIMATES OF INDIVIDUAL RISK

The clinical meaning attached to relative and attributable risk is often quite different, because the two expressions of risk stand for entirely different concepts. The appropriate expression of risk depends on which question is being asked.

> *Example* Risk factors for cardiovascular disease are generally thought to be weaker among the elderly than the middle-aged. This assertion was examined by comparing the relative risks and attributable risks of common risk factors for cardiovascular disease among different age groups (8). An example is the risk of stroke from smoking (Table 5.5). The relative risk decreases with age, from 4.0 in persons ages 45–49 to 1.4 in persons aged 65–69. However, the attributable risk increases slightly with age, mainly because stroke is more common in the elderly regardless of smoking status. Thus, although the causal link between smoking and stroke decreases with age, an elderly individual who smokes increases his or her actual risk of stroke to a similar, indeed slightly greater, degree than a younger person.

Table 5.5
Comparing Relative Risk and Attributable Risk in the Relationship of Smoking, Stroke, and Age[a]

Age	Incidence (per 1000)		Relative Risk	Attributable Risk
	Nonsmokers	Smokers		
45–49	7.4	29.7	4.0	22.3
50–54	17.2	37.0	2.2	19.8
55–59	27.9	64.7	2.3	36.7
60–64	47.4	76.9	1.6	29.5
65–69	80.2	110.4	1.4	30.2

[a] Adapted from Psaty BM et al. J Clin Epidemiol 1990;43:961–970.

In most clinical situations, because attributable risk represents the actual additional probability of disease in those exposed, it is a more meaningful expression of risk for individuals than is relative risk. On the other hand, relative risk is more useful for expressing the strength of a causal relationship.

POPULATION RISK

Another way of looking at risk is to ask, "How much does a risk factor contribute to the overall rates of disease in groups of people, rather than individuals?" This information is useful for deciding which risk factors are particularly important and which are trivial to the overall health of a community, and so it can inform those in policy positions how to choose priorities for the deployment of health care resources. A relatively weak risk factor (i.e., one with a small relative risk) that is quite prevalent in a community could account for more disease than a very strong, but rare, risk factor.

To estimate population risk, it is necessary to take into account the frequency with which members of a community are exposed to a risk factor. *Population attributable risk* is the product of the attributable risk and the prevalence of the risk factor in a population. It measures the excess incidence of disease in a community that is associated with a risk factor. One can also describe the fraction of disease occurrence in a population that is associated with a particular risk factor, the *population attributable fraction*. It is obtained by dividing the population attributable risk by the total incidence of disease in the population.

Figure 5.4 illustrates how the prevalence of a risk factor determines the relationship between individual and population risk. Figure 5.4*A* shows the attributable risk of death according to diastolic blood pressure. Risk increases with increasing blood pressure. However, few people have extremely high blood pressure (Fig. 5.4*B*). When hypertension is defined as

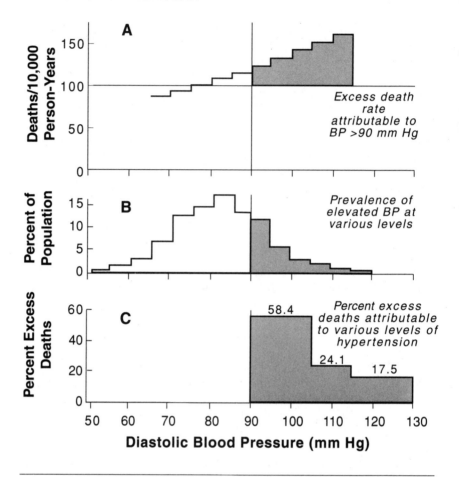

Figure 5.4. Relationships among attributable risk, prevalence of risk factor, and population risk for hypertension. (Adapted from The Hypertension Detection and Follow-up Cooperative Group. Mild hypertensives in the hypertension detection and follow-up program. Ann N Y Acad Sci 1978;304:254–266.)

having a diastolic blood pressure >90 mm Hg, most hypertensive people are just over 90 mm Hg, and very few are in the highest category (≥115 mm Hg). As a result, the greatest percentage of excess deaths in the population (58.4%) is attributable to relatively low-grade hypertension, 90–105 mm Hg (Fig. 5.4C). Paradoxically, then, physicians could save more lives by effective treatment of mild hypertension than severe hypertension. This fact, so counterintuitive to clinical thinking, has been termed "the prevention paradox" (9).

Measures of population risk are less frequently encountered in the clinical literature than are measures of individual risk, e.g., attributable and relative risks. But a particular clinical practice is as much a population for the doctor as is a community for health policymakers. Also, how the prevalence of exposure affects community risk can be important in the care of individual patients. For instance, when patients cannot give a history or when exposure is difficult for them to recognize, we depend on the usual prevalence of exposure to estimate the likelihood of various diseases. When considering treatable causes of cirrhosis in a North American patient, for example, it would be more profitable to consider alcohol than schistosomes, inasmuch as few North Americans are exposed to *Schistosoma mansoni*. Of course, one might take a very different stance in the Nile delta, where schistosomes are prevalent and the people, who are mostly Muslims, rarely drink alcohol.

Summary

Risk factors are characteristics that are associated with an increased risk of becoming diseased. Whether or not a particular risk factor is a cause of disease, its presence allows one to predict the probability that disease will occur.

Most suspected risk factors cannot be manipulated for the purposes of an experiment, so it is usually necessary to study risk by simply observing people's experience with risk factors and disease. One way of doing so is to select a cohort of people, some members of which are and some of which are not exposed to a risk factor, and observe the subsequent incidence of disease. Although it is scientifically preferable to study risk by means of cohort studies, this approach is not always feasible because of the time, effort, and expense it entails.

When disease rates are compared among groups with different exposures to a risk factor, the results can be expressed in several ways. Attributable risk is the excess incidence of disease related to exposure. Relative risk is the number of times more likely exposed people are to become diseased relative to nonexposed people. The impact of a risk factor on groups of people takes into account not only the risk related to exposure but the prevalence of exposure as well.

REFERENCES

1. Weiss NS, Liff JM. Accounting for the multicausal nature of disease in the design and analysis of epidemiologic studies. Am J Epidemiol 1983;117:14–18.
2. Prabhat KSJ, Beral V, Peto J, Hack S, Hermon C, Deacon J. Antibodies to human papillomavirus and to other genital infectious agents and invasive cervical cancer risk. Lancet 1993;341:1116–1118.
3. Rose G. Sick individuals and sick populations. Int J Epidemiol 1985;14:32–38.
4. Diamond GA, Forrester JS. Analysis of probability as an aid in the clinical diagnosis of coronary-artery disease. N Engl J Med 1979;300:1350–1358.

5. Jaffe HW et al. National case-control study of Kaposi's sarcoma and *Pneumocystis carinii* pneumonia in homosexual men. Part 1, Epidemiologic results. Ann Intern Med 1983;99:145–151.
6. Dawber TR. The Framingham Study. The epidemiology of atherosclerotic disease. Cambridge, MA: Harvard University Press, 1980.
7. Kramer MS, Rooks Y, Pearson HA. Growth and development in children with sickle-cell trait. N Engl J Med 1978;299:686–689.
8. Psaty BM et al. Risk ratios and risk differences in estimating the effect of risk factors for cardiovascular disease in the elderly. J Clin Epidemiol 1990;43:961–970.
9. Hofman A, Vandenbroucke JP. Geoffrey Rose's big idea. Br Med J 1992;305:1519–1520.

SUGGESTED READINGS

Detsky AS, O'Rourke K, Corey PN, Johnston N, Fenton S, Jeejeebhoy KN. The hazards of using active clinic patients as a source of subjects for clinical studies. J Gen Intern Med 1988;3:260–266.

Feinstein AR. Scientific standards in epidemiologic studies of the menace of daily life. Science 1988;242:1257–1263. Response by Savitz DA, Greenland S, Stolley PD, Kelsey JL. Scientific standards of criticism: a reaction to "Scientific standards in epidemiologic studies of the menace of daily life" by Feinstein. Epidemiology 1990;1:78–83.

Malenka DJ, Baron JA, Johansen S, Wahrenberger JW, Ross JM. The framing effect of relative and absolute risk. J Gen Intern Med 1993;8:543–548.

Morganstern H, Kleinbaum DG, Kupper LL. Measures of disease incidence used in epidemiologic research. Int J Epidemiol 1980;9:97–104.

Naylor CD, Chen E, Strauss B. Measured enthusiasm: does the method of reporting trial results alter perceptions of therapeutic effectiveness? Ann Intern Med 1992;117:916–921.

6

PROGNOSIS

When people become sick, they have a great many questions about how their illness will affect them. Is it dangerous? Could I die of it? Will there be pain? How long will I be able to continue my present activities? Will it ever go away altogether? Most patients and their families want to know what to expect, even if little can be done about their illness.

Prognosis is a prediction of the future course of disease following its onset. In this chapter, we review the ways in which the course of disease can be described. We then consider the biases that can affect these descriptions and how these biases can be controlled. Our intention is to give readers a better understanding of a difficult but indispensable task—predicting patients' futures as closely as possible. The object is to avoid expressing prognosis with vagueness when it is unnecessary, and with certainty when it is misleading.

Doctors and patients think about prognosis in several different ways. First, they want to know the general course of the illness the patient has. A young patient suffering from postherpetic neuralgia associated with herpes zoster can be assured that the pain usually resolves in less than a month. Second, they usually want to know, as much as possible, the prognosis in the particular case. Even though HIV infection is virtually universally fatal, individuals with the infection may live from a few months to more than a decade; a patient wants to know where on this continuum his or her particular case falls. Third, patients especially are interested to know how an illness is likely to affect their lives, not only whether it will or will not kill them, but how it will change their ability to work, to walk, to talk, how it will alter their relationships with family and friends, how much pain and discomfort they will have to endure.

Prognosis Studies

Studies of prognosis tackle these clinical questions in ways similar to cohort studies of risk. A group of patients having something in common (a particular medical disease or condition, in the case of prognostic studies)

111

are assembled and followed forward in time, and clinical outcomes are measured. Often, conditions that are associated with a given outcome of the disease, i.e., *prognostic factors*, are sought.

CLINICAL COURSE/NATURAL HISTORY OF DISEASE

Disease prognosis can be described for either the clinical course or the natural history of illness. The term *clinical course* has been used to describe the evolution (prognosis) of disease that has come under medical care and is then treated in a variety of ways that might affect the subsequent course of events. Patients usually come under medical care at some time in the course of their illness when they have diseases that cause symptoms such as pain, failure to thrive, disfigurement, or unusual behavior. Examples include type I diabetes mellitus, carcinoma of the lung, and rabies. Once disease is recognized, it is also likely to be treated.

The prognosis of disease without medical intervention is termed the *natural history* of disease. Natural history describes how patients will fare if nothing is done for their disease. A great many medical conditions, even in countries with advanced medical care systems, often do not come under medical care. They remain unrecognized, perhaps because they are asymptomatic or are considered among the ordinary discomforts of daily living. Examples include mild depression, anemia, and cancers that are occult and slow growing (e.g., some cancers of the thyroid and prostate).

ZERO TIME

Cohorts in prognostic studies are observed starting from a point in time, called *zero time*. This point should be specified clearly and be the same well-defined location along the course of disease (e.g., the onset of symptoms, time of diagnosis, or beginning of treatment) for each patient. The term *inception cohort* is used to describe a group of people who are assembled near the onset (inception) of disease.

If observation is begun at different points in the course of disease for the various patients in the cohort, description of their subsequent course will lack precision. The relative timing of such events as recovery, recurrence, and death would be difficult to interpret or misleading.

For example, suppose we wanted to describe the clinical course of patients with lung cancer. We would assemble a cohort of people with the disease and follow them forward over time to such outcomes as complications and death. But what do we mean by "with disease"? If zero time was detection by screening for some patients, onset of symptoms for others, and hospitalization or the beginning of treatment for still others, then observed prognosis would depend on the particular mix of zero times in the study. Worse, if we did not explicitly describe when in the course of disease patients entered the cohort, we would not know how to interpret or use the reported prognosis.

DESCRIBING OUTCOMES OF DISEASE

Descriptions of prognosis should include the full range of manifestations that would be considered important to patients. This means not only death and disease but also consequences of disease such as pain, anguish, and inability to care for one's self or pursue usual activities. (The Five Ds listed in Table 1.2 are a simple way to summarize important clinical outcomes.)

In their efforts to be "scientific," physicians sometimes value certain kinds of outcomes over others, at the expense of clinical relevance. Clinical effects that cannot be directly perceived by patients (e.g., reduction in tumor size, normalization of blood chemistries, or change in serology) are not ends in themselves. It is appropriate to substitute these biologic phenomena for clinical outcomes only if the two are known to be related to each other. Thus hypercalcemia is an important clinical outcome of hyperparathyroidism only if it causes symptoms such as drowsiness or thirst or if there is reason to believe that it will eventually lead to complications such as bone or kidney disease. If an outcome cannot be related to something patients will recognize, the information should not be used to guide patient care, although it may be of considerable value in understanding the origins and mechanisms of disease.

HEALTH-RELATED QUALITY-OF-LIFE MEASURES

There is growing recognition that "health" involves more than the avoidance of negative aspects such as death and disease. Clinical activities should have a positive impact on how a person functions and lives. This concept has been referred to as *health-related quality of life, health status,* or *functional status.* Questionnaires have been developed to measure patients' quality of life. Sometimes their use strengthens arguments for certain clinical interventions. For example, a study showed that erythropoietin treatment of patients with chronic renal failure not only increased patients' hematocrits but improved their health-related quality of life (1). On the other hand, sometimes quality-of-life measurements reveal complicated trade-offs. A study of zidovudine (AZT) treatment in patients with mildly symptomatic HIV infection showed that although the drug delayed progression to AIDS by an average of 0.9 months, the positive result was offset by adverse effects of the drug. Thus patients receiving the drug had an average of 14.5 months without disease progression or severe symptomatic adverse effects from AZT compared with an average of 14.7 months for patients not receiving the drug (2). What looked like a small benefit in delayed progression to AIDS was not so clear when quality-of-life measures were added to the study.

Prognostic Factors

Although most patients are interested in the course of their disease in general, they are even more interested in a prediction for their given case. *Prognostic factors* help identify groups of patients with the same disease who have different prognoses.

DIFFERENCES BETWEEN PROGNOSTIC FACTORS AND RISK FACTORS

Studies of risk factors usually deal with healthy people, whereas prognostic factors—conditions that are associated with an outcome of disease—are, by definition, studied in sick people. There are other important differences as well, outlined below.

Different Factors

Factors associated with an increased risk are not necessarily the same as those marking a worse prognosis and are often considerably different for a given disease. For example, low blood pressure decreases one's chances of having an acute myocardial infarction, but it is a bad prognostic sign when present during the acute event (Fig. 6.1). Similarly, intake of exogenous estrogens during menopause increases women's risk of endometrial cancer, but the associated cancers are found at an earlier stage and seem to have a better-than-average prognosis.

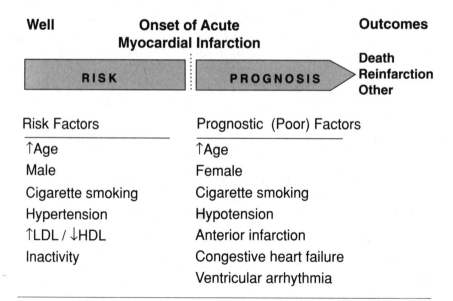

Risk Factors	Prognostic (Poor) Factors
↑Age	↑Age
Male	Female
Cigarette smoking	Cigarette smoking
Hypertension	Hypotension
↑LDL / ↓HDL	Anterior infarction
Inactivity	Congestive heart failure
	Ventricular arrhythmia

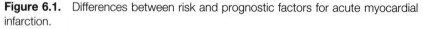

Figure 6.1. Differences between risk and prognostic factors for acute myocardial infarction.

Some factors do have a similar effect on both risk and prognosis. For example, both the risk of experiencing an acute myocardial infarction and the risk of dying of it increase with age.

Different Outcomes

Risk and prognosis describe different phenomena. For risk, the event being counted is the onset of disease. For prognosis, a variety of consequences of disease are counted, including death, complications, disability, and suffering.

Different Rates

Risk factors generally predict low probability events. Yearly rates for the onset of various diseases are on the order of 1/100 to 1/10,000. As a result, relationships between exposure and risk usually elude even astute clinicians unless they rely on carefully executed studies, often involving a large number of people over extended periods of time. Prognosis, on the other hand, describes relatively frequent events. Clinicians often can form good estimates of prognosis on their own, from their personal experience. For example, they know that few patients with lung or pancreatic cancer survive as long as 5 years, whereas most with chronic lymphocytic leukemia survive much longer.

MULTIPLE PROGNOSTIC FACTORS AND PREDICTION RULES

A combination of factors may give a more precise prognosis than each of the same factors taken one at a time. *Clinical prediction rules* estimate the probability of outcomes according to a set of patient characteristics.

> *Example*   Once patients with HIV infection develop AIDS, the prognosis is poor and survival time is short. Even so, and before antiviral and prophylactic therapy for opportunistic infections became standard treatment, it was clear that some patients with AIDS survived much longer than others. A study was done to determine which patient characteristics predicted survival (3). Each of several physiologic characteristics was found to be related to survival. Using these factors in combination, the investigators developed a prognostic staging system, with 1 point for the presence of each of 7 factors: severe diarrhea or a serum albumin <2.0 gm/dL, any neurologic deficit, PO_2 less than or equal to 50 mm Hg, hematocrit <30%, lymphocyte count <150/mL, white count <2500/mL, and platelet count <140,000/mL. The total score determined the prognostic stage (I, 0 points; II, 1 point; III, greater than or equal to 2 points). Figure 6.2 shows the survival of AIDS patients in each prognostic stage. Using multiple prognostic factors together, the authors noted that prediction for median length of survival varied from 11.5 months for patients in stage I to 2.1 months for patients in stage III.

Describing Prognosis

PROGNOSIS AS A RATE

It is convenient to summarize the course of disease as a single number, or *rate:* the proportion of people experiencing an event. Rates commonly

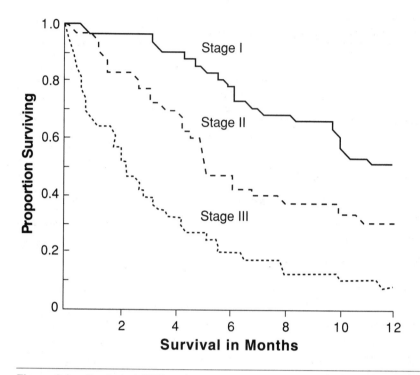

Figure 6.2. Survival of AIDS patients according to prognostic stage. Median survival times (in months): stage I, 11.6; stage II, 5.1; stage III, 2.1. (Adapted from Justice AC, Feinstein AR, Wells CK. A new prognostic staging system for the acquired immunodeficiency syndrome. N Eng J Med 1989;320:1388–1393.)

used for this purpose are shown in Table 6.1. These rates have in common the same basic components of incidence, events arising in a cohort of patients over time.

All the components of the rate must be specified: zero time, the specific clinical characteristics of the patients, definition of outcome events, and length of follow-up. Follow-up must be long enough for all the events to occur; otherwise, the observed rate will understate the true one.

A TRADE-OFF: SIMPLICITY VERSUS MORE INFORMATION

Expressing prognosis as a rate has the virtue of simplicity. Rates can be committed to memory and communicated succinctly. Their drawback is that relatively little information is conveyed, and large differences in prognosis can be hidden within similar summary rates.

Figure 6.3 shows 5-year survival for patients with four conditions. For each condition, about 10% of the patients are alive at 5 years. But similar

Table 6.1
Rates Commonly Used to Describe Prognosis

Rate	Definition[a]
5-year survival	Percent of patients surviving 5 years from some point in the course of their disease
Case fatality	Percent of patients with a disease who die of it
Disease-specific mortality	Number of people per 10,000 (or 100,000) population dying of a specific disease
Response	Percent of patients showing some evidence of improvement following an intervention
Remission	Percent of patients entering a phase in which disease is no longer detectable
Recurrence	Percent of patients who have return of disease after a disease-free interval

[a] Time under observation is either stated or assumed to be sufficiently long so that all events that will occur have been observed.

summary rates of approximately 10% survival obscure differences of considerable importance to patients. Early survival in patients with dissecting aneurysms is very poor, but if they survive the first few months, their risk of dying is not affected by having had the aneurysm (Fig. 6.3*A*). On the other hand, HIV positive patients who develop AIDS die throughout the 5 years (Fig. 6.3*B*). Chronic granulocytic leukemia is a condition that has relatively little effect on survival during the first few years after diagnosis (Fig. 6.3*C*). Later, there is an acceleration in mortality rate until nearly all patients are dead 5 years after diagnosis. Figure 6.3*D* is presented as a benchmark. Only at age 100 do people in the general population have a 5-year survival rate comparable to that of patients with the three diseases.

SURVIVAL ANALYSIS

When interpreting prognosis, we would like to know the likelihood, on the average, that patients with a given condition will experience an outcome at any point in time. When prognosis is expressed as a summary rate it does not contain this information. However, there are methods for presenting information about average time to event for any point in the course of disease.

SURVIVAL OF A COHORT

The most straightforward way to learn about survival is to assemble a cohort of patients with the condition of interest at some point in the course of their illness (e.g., onset of symptoms, diagnosis, or beginning of treatment) and keep them under observation until all could have experienced the outcome of interest. For a small cohort, one might then represent the experience with these patients' course of disease as shown in Figure 6.4*A*.

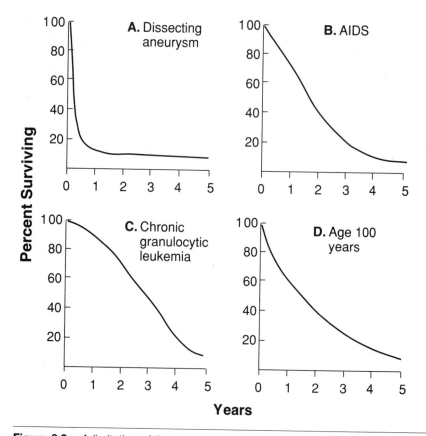

Figure 6.3. A limitation of 5-year survival rates: four conditions with the same 5-year survival rate of 10%. (Data from Anagnostopoulos CD et al. Aortic dissections and dissecting aneurysms. Am J Cardiology 1972;30:263–273; Saah JA, Hoover DR et al. Factors influencing survival after AIDS: report from the Multicenter AIDS Cohort Study (MACS). J Acquir Immune Defic Syndr 1994;7:287–295; Kardinal CG et al. Chronic granulocytic leukemia. Review of 536 cases. Arch Intern Med 1976;136:305–313; and American College of Life Insurance. 1979 life insurance fact book. Washington, DC: ACLI 1979.)

The plot of survival against time displays steps, corresponding to the death of each of the 10 patients in the cohort. If the number of patients were increased (Fig. 6.4B), the size of the steps would diminish. If a very large number of patients were represented, the figure would approximate a smooth curve. This information could then be used to predict the year-by-year, or even week-by-week, prognosis of similar patients.

Unfortunately, obtaining the information in this way is impractical for several reasons. Some of the patients would undoubtedly drop out of the study before the end of the follow-up period, perhaps because of another illness, a move to a place where follow-up was impractical, or dissatisfaction with the study. These patients would have to be excluded from the cohort, even though considerable effort may have been exerted to gather data on them up to the point at which they dropped out. Also, it would be necessary to wait until all of the cohort's members had reached each point in time before the probability of surviving to that point could be calculated. Because patients ordinarily become available for a study over a period of time, at any point in calendar time there would be a relatively long follow-up for patients who entered the study first, but only brief experience with those who entered recently. The last patient who entered the study would have to reach each year of follow-up before any information on survival to that year would be available.

SURVIVAL CURVES

To make efficient use of all available data from each patient in the cohort, a way of estimating the survival of a cohort over time, called *survival analysis,* has been developed. (The usual method is called a Kaplan-Meir analysis, after the originators.) The purpose of survival analysis is not (as its name implies) only to describe whether patients live or die. Any outcome that is dichotomous and occurs only once during follow-up— e.g., time to coronary event or to recurrence of cancer—can be described in this way. When an event other than survival is described, the term *time-to-event analysis* is sometimes used.

Figure 6.5 shows a typical survival curve. On the vertical axis is the

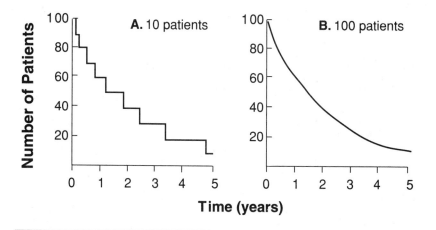

Figure 6.4. Survival of two cohorts, small and large, when all members are observed for the full period of follow-up.

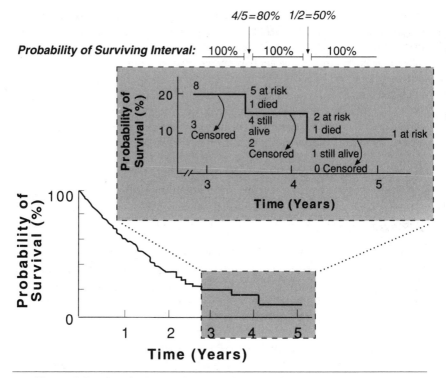

Figure 6.5.   A typical survival curve, with detail for one part of the curve.

probability of surviving, and on the horizontal axis is the period of time following the beginning of observation. Often, the numbers of patients at risk at various points in time are shown to give some idea of the contribution of chance to the observed rates.

The probability of surviving to any point in time is estimated from the cumulative probability of surviving each of the time intervals that preceded it. Time intervals can be made as small as necessary; in Kaplan-Meir analyses, the intervals are between each new event (death) and the preceding one. Most of the time, no one dies, and the probability of surviving is 1. When one or more patients die, the probability of surviving is calculated as the ratio of the number of patients surviving to the number at risk of dying at that time. Patients who have already died, dropped out, or have not yet been followed-up to that point are not at risk of dying and so are not used to estimate survival for that time. When patients are lost from the study at any point in time, for any reason, they are *censored*, i.e., they are no longer counted in the denominator. The probability of surviving does not change during intervals in which no one dies; so in practice, the probability of surviving is recalculated only for times when there is a death. Although the probability assigned at any given interval is not very accurate, because of the small number of events involved, the overall probability of surviving up to each point in time (which is the product of all preceding probabilities) is remarkably accurate.

A part of the survival curve in Figure 6.5 (from 3 to 5 years after zero time) is presented in detail to illustrate the data used to estimate survival: patients at risk, patients no longer at risk (censored), and patients experiencing outcome events at each point in time.

INTERPRETING SURVIVAL CURVES

Several points must be kept in mind when interpreting survival curves. First, the vertical axis represents the estimated probability of surviving for members of a hypothetical cohort, not the percent surviving for an actual cohort.

Second, points on a survival curve are the best estimate, for a given set of data, of the probability of survival for members of a cohort. However, the precision of these estimates depends, as do all observations on samples, on the number of observations on which the estimate is based. One can be more confident that the estimates on the left-hand side of the curve are sound, because more patients are at risk during this time. But at the tail of the curve, on the right, the number of patients on whom estimates of survival are based often becomes relatively small because deaths, dropouts, and late entrants to the study result in fewer and fewer patients being followed for that length of time. As a result, estimates of survival toward the end of the follow-up period are imprecise and can be strongly affected by what happens to relatively few patients. For example, in Figure 6.5, the probability of surviving is 8% at 5 years. If at that point the one remaining patient happens to die, the probability of surviving would fall to zero. Clearly, this would be a too literal reading of the data. Estimates of survival at the tails of survival curves must, therefore, be interpreted with caution.

Finally, the shape of some survival curves, particularly those in which most patients experience the event of interest, gives the impression that the event occurs more frequently early on than later, when the slope reaches a plateau and it appears that the risk of outcome events is considerably less. But this impression is deceptive. As time passes, rates of survival are being applied to a diminishing number of people, causing the slope of the curve to flatten even when the rate of outcome events does not change.

Variations on the basic survival curve are found in the medical literature (Fig. 6.6). Often the proportion with, rather than without, the outcome event is indicated on the vertical axis; the curve then sweeps upward and to the right. Other variations increase the amount of information presented with the curve. The number of patients at risk at various points in time

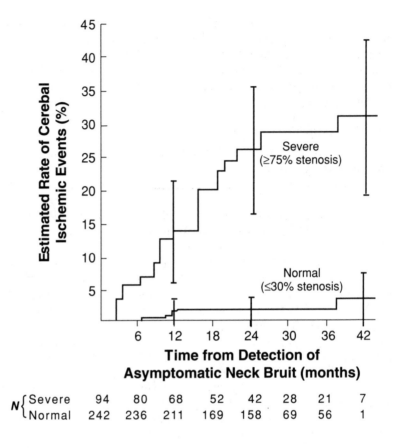

Figure 6.6. Survival curve showing comparison of two cohorts, number of people at risk, and 95% confidence intervals for observed rates. These curves show the cumulative probability of a cerebral ischemic event from time of diagnosis, according to the initial degree of carotid stenosis. (Data from Chambers BR, Norris, JW. Outcome in patients with asymptomatic neck bruits. N Engl J Med 1986;315:860–865.)

can be included under the horizontal axis; the precision of estimates of survival, which declines with time because fewer and fewer patients are still under observation as time passes, can be identified by confidence intervals (see Chapter 9); and survival curves for patients with different characteristics (e.g., patients with different prognostic factors or treatments) can be compared in the same figure. Sometimes tics (not shown in Fig. 6.6) are added to the survival curves, to indicate each time a patient is censored.

Survival curves can be constructed for combinations of prognostic factors. This can be done by stratifying patients according to the presence or absence of a set of prognostic factors, as shown earlier in this chapter. A statistical technique called the *Cox proportional hazards regression model* can be used to identify a combination of factors that best predicts prognosis in the group of patients under study or the effect of individual factors independently (Chapter 9).

Bias in Cohort Studies

Potential for bias exists in any observation. Bias in cohort studies— whether to study risk or prognosis—can create apparent differences when they do not actually exist in nature or obscure differences when they really do exist.

Bias can be recognized more easily when one knows where it is most likely to occur in the course of a study. First, it is important to determine if bias could be present under the conditions of the study. Second, determine if bias is actually present in the particular study being considered. Third, decide if the consequences of bias are sufficiently large that they distort the conclusions in a clinically important way. If damage to the study's conclusions is not very great, then the presence of bias will not lead to misleading results. Some of the characteristic locations of bias in cohort research are illustrated in Figure 6.7 and described below.

SUSCEPTIBILITY BIAS

A form of selection bias, called *susceptibility bias,* occurs when groups of patients assembled for study differ in ways other than the factors under study. These extraneous factors, not the particular factors being studied, may determine the outcome. A comparable term is *assembly bias.* Groups

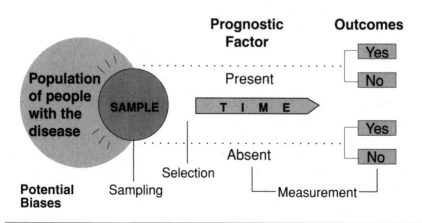

Figure 6.7. Locations of potential bias in cohort studies.

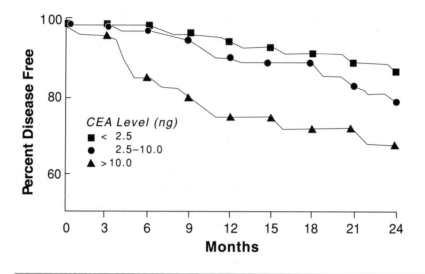

Figure 6.8.   Disease-free survival according to CEA levels in colorectal cancer patients with similar pathological staging (Dukes B). (Redrawn from Wolmark N et al. The prognostic significance of preoperative carcinoembryonic antigen levels in colorectal cancer. Results from NSABP clinical trials. Ann Surg 1984;199:375–382.)

being compared are not equally susceptible to the outcome of interest, other than the factor under study.

Susceptibility bias in prognosis studies may be due to one or more differences among cohorts, including the extent of disease, the presence of other diseases, the point of time in the course of disease, and prior treatment. The following illustrates how susceptibility bias was assessed in a study of the prognostic value of carcinoembryonic antigen results in patients with colorectal cancer.

> *Example*   Increased levels of carcinoembryonic antigen (CEA), a tumor-associated fetal antigen, are found in several types of tumors, including colorectal cancer. A study was undertaken to determine if preoperative CEA levels predict relapse of disease after surgical resection with the intent to cure (4). CEA levels were found to correlate with the extent of disease (frequently categorized according to "Dukes classification": A, tumors confined to the bowel wall; B, tumors extending through the bowel wall but not to the lymph nodes; C, tumors involving regional lymph nodes; and D, tumors having distant metastases). Mean CEA levels varied with extent of disease: 4 for Dukes A, 9 for B, 32 for C, and 251 for D. Both Dukes classification and CEA level strongly predicted disease relapse. But did the CEA level predict independently of the Dukes classification or was susceptibility of relapse explained by Dukes classification alone? To answer this question, the association of preoperative CEA levels to disease relapse was examined for patients in each Dukes classification. Figure 6.8 shows that for Dukes B classification,

CEA levels independently predicted relapse. Similar results were found for patients with Dukes C tumors. Therefore, the association between CEA levels and likelihood of relapse could not be explained by susceptibility bias for patients with Dukes B and C colorectal cancers, and CEA is an important independent prognostic factor.

SURVIVAL COHORTS

True cohort studies should be distinguished from studies of *survival cohorts* in which patients are included in a study because they both have a disease and are currently available—perhaps because they are being seen in a specialized clinic. Another term for such groups of patients is *available patient cohorts*. Reports of survival cohorts are misleading if they are presented as true cohorts. In a survival cohort, people are assembled at various times in the course of their disease, rather than at the beginning, as in a true cohort study. Their clinical course is then described by going back in time and seeing how they have fared up to the present (Fig. 6.9). The experiences of survival cohorts are sometimes presented as if they

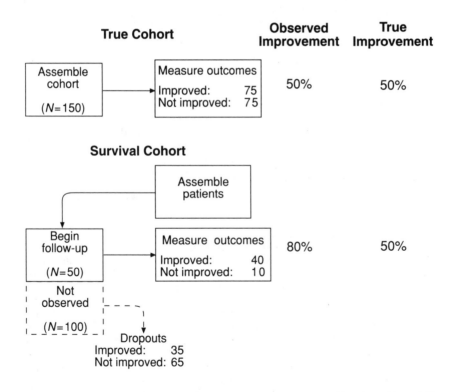

Figure 6.9. Comparison of a true and a "survival" cohort; in the survival cohort, some of the patients present at the beginning are not included in the follow-up.

were descriptions of the course of disease from its inception. However, they may represent a biased view, because they include only those patients who are available for study some time after their disease began. For lethal conditions, the patients in a survival cohort are the ones who are fortunate enough to have survived and so are available for observation years later. For diseases that remit, the patients are the ones who are unfortunate enough to have persistent disease. In effect, survival cohorts describe the past history of prevalent cases and not what one would expect over the time following the onset of disease. Thus a survival cohort is a special case of assembly bias.

Reports of survival cohorts are relatively common in the medical literature, particularly in the form of "case series" (discussed in Chapter 10). Such reports can make an important contribution, primarily by describing early experiences with newly defined syndromes, but they represent tentative, not conclusive, observations.

> ***Example*** Concern has been raised about the possibility that silicone breast implants may cause autoimmune symptoms of rheumatic disease. A study was, therefore, done of 156 women with silicone breast implants and rheumatic disease complaints (5). The patients were consecutive referrals to three rheumatologists who were known for their interest in silicone implants and rheumatic disease. Serologic tests in the women were compared to those of women without implants but with fibromyalgia and to tests in women with implants but no rheumatic symptoms. The clinical findings in the women with implants and complaints were described; most did not fulfill criteria for rheumatoid arthritis and most had normal immunologic tests. However, 14 patients had scleroderma-like illness and abnormal serology that was not found in the comparison groups. Because of the possible biases that can occur in the assembly of patients for this case series, the authors were cautious about their findings, concluding that "the hypotheses raised in this study and others should be tested in large, population-based studies." Publication of the first such study does not support the hypothesis (6).

MIGRATION BIAS

Migration bias, another form of selection bias, can occur when patients in one group leave their original group, dropping out of the study altogether or moving to one of the other groups under study. If these changes take place on a sufficiently large scale, they can affect the validity of conclusions.

In nearly all studies, some members of an original group drop out over time. If these dropouts occur randomly, such that the characteristics of lost subjects in one group are on the average similar to those lost from the other, then no bias would be introduced. This is so whether or not the number of dropouts is large or the number is similar in the groups. But ordinarily the characteristics of lost subjects are not the same in various groups. The reasons for dropping out—death, recovery, side effects of treatment, etc.—are often related to prognosis and may also affect one group more than another. As a result, groups in a cohort that were comparable at the outset may become less so as time passes.

As the proportion of people in the cohort who are not followed up increases, the potential for bias increases. It is not difficult to estimate how large this bias could be. All one needs is the number of people in the cohort, the number not accounted for, and the observed outcome rate.

> *Example* Thompson et al. described the long-term outcomes of gastro-gastrostomy (7). A cohort of 123 morbidly obese patients was studied 19–47 months after surgery. Success was defined as having lost more than 30% of excess weight.
>
> Only 103 patients (84%) could be located. In these, the success rate of surgery was 60/103 (58%). To determine the range within which the true success rate must lie, the authors did a *best case/worst case analysis*. Success rates were calculated, assuming that all of the patients lost to follow-up were, on the one hand, successes (best case) and, on the other hand, failures (worst case). Of the total cohort of 123 patients, 103 were followed up and 20 were lost to follow-up. The observed success rate was 60/103, or 58%. In the best case, all 20 patients lost to follow-up would be counted as successes, and the success rate would be (60 + 20)/123, or 65%. In the worst case, all 20 patients would be counted as failures, and the success rate would be 60/123, or 49%. Thus the true rate must have been between 49 and 65%; probably, it was closer to 58%, the observed rate, because patients not followed up are unlikely to be all successes or all failures.

Patients may also cross over from one group to another in the cohort during their follow-up. Whenever this occurs, the original reasons for patients being in one group or the other no longer apply. If exchange of patients between groups takes place on a large scale, it can diminish the observed difference in risk compared to what might have been observed if the original groups had remained intact. Migration bias due to crossover is more often a problem in risk than in prognosis studies, because risk studies often go on for many years. On the other hand, migration from one group to another can be used in the analysis of a study.

> *Example* The relationship between lifestyle and mortality was studied by classifying 10,269 Harvard College alumni by physical activity, smoking status, weight, and blood pressure in 1966 and again in 1977 (8). Mortality rates were then observed over a 9-year period from 1977 to 1985. It was recognized that original classifications might change, obscuring any relationship that might exist between lifestyle and mortality. To deal with this, the investigators defined four categories: men who maintained high-risk lifestyles, those who changed from low- to high-risk lifestyles, those who changed from high- to low-risk lifestyles, and those who maintained low-risk lifestyles. After adjusting for other risk factors, men who increased their physical activity from low to moderate amounts, quit smoking, lost weight to normal levels, and/or became normotensive all had lower mortality than men who maintained or adopted high-risk characteristics, but not as low as the rates for alumni who never had any risk factors.

MEASUREMENT BIAS

Measurement bias is possible if patients in one group stand a better chance of having their outcome detected than those in another group. Obviously, some outcomes, such as death, cardiovascular catastrophes, and major cancers, are so obtrusive that they are unlikely to be missed. But for less clear-cut outcomes—the specific cause of death, subclinical disease, side effects, or disability—measurement bias can occur because of differences in the methods with which the outcome is sought or classified.

Measurement bias can be minimized in three general ways. One can ensure that those who make the observations are unaware of the group to which each patient belongs, can set careful rules for deciding whether or not an outcome event has occurred (and follow the rules), and can apply efforts to discover events equally in all groups in the study.

> **Example** Chambers and Norris studied the outcome of patients with asymptomatic neck bruits (9). A total of 500 asymptomatic patients with cervical bruits were observed for up to 4 years. Patients were classified according to the degree of initial carotid artery stenosis by Doppler ultrasonography. Outcomes were change in degree of carotid stenosis and incidence of cerebral ischemic events.
>
> To avoid biased measurements, the authors estimated carotid stenosis using established, explicit criteria for interpreting Doppler scans and made the readings without knowledge of the auscultatory or previous Doppler findings. Clinical and Doppler assessments were repeated every 6 months, and all noncomplying patients were telephoned to determine whether outcomes had occurred.
>
> This study showed, among other things, that patients with >75% carotid stenosis had a >20% incidence of cerebral ischemic events in 3 years, more than 4 times the rate of patients with <30% stenosis (see Fig. 6.6).

Dealing with Selection Bias

To determine how a factor is related to prognosis, ideally we would like to compare cohorts with and without the factor, everything else being equal. But in real life "everything else" is usually not equal in cohort studies.

What can be done about this problem? There are several possible ways of *controlling* for differences during either designing or analyzing research (Table 6.2).[1] For any observational study, if one or more of these strategies have not been applied, the reader should be skeptical. The basic question is, "Are the differences in prognosis in the groups related to the particular factor under study or to some other factor(s)?"

---

[1] *Control* has several meanings in research: (a) general term for any process—restriction, matching, stratification, adjustment—aimed at removing the effects of extraneous variables while examining the independent effects of one variable, (b) the nonexposed people in a cohort study (a confusing use of the term), (c) the nontreated patients in a clinical trial, and (d) nondiseased people (noncases) in a case control study (see Chapter 10).

Table 6.2
Methods for Controlling Selection Bias

Method	Description	Phase of Study	
		Design	Analysis
Randomization	Assign patients to groups in a way that gives each patient an equal chance of falling into one or the other group	+	
Restriction	Limit the range of characteristics of patients in the study	+	
Matching	For each patient in one group, select one or more patients with the same characteristics (except for the one under study) for a comparison group	+	
Stratification	Compare rates within subgroups (strata) with otherwise similar probability of the outcome		+
Adjustment			
Simple	Mathematically adjust crude rates for one or a few characteristics so that equal weight is given to strata of similar risk		+
Multiple	Adjust for differences in a large number of factors related to outcome, using mathematical modeling techniques		+
Best case/ worst case	Describe how different the results could be under the most extreme (or simply very unlikely) conditions of selection bias		+

RANDOMIZATION

The only way to equalize all extraneous factors, or "everything else," is to assign patients to groups randomly so that each patient has an equal chance of falling into the exposed or unexposed group. A special feature of randomization is that it not only equalizes factors we think might affect prognosis, it also equalizes factors we do not know about. Thus randomization goes a long way in protecting us from incorrect conclusions about prognostic factors. However, it is usually not possible to study prognosis in this way. The special situations in which it is possible to allocate exposure randomly, usually to study the effects of treatment on prognosis, will be discussed in Chapter 7.

RESTRICTION

Patients who are enrolled in a study can be restricted to only those possessing a narrow range of characteristics, to equalize important extraneous factors. For example, the effect of age on prognosis after acute myocardial infarction could be studied in white males with uncomplicated anterior myocardial infarctions. However, one should keep in mind that although restriction on entry to a study can certainly produce homogeneous groups of patients, it does so at the expense of generalizability. In the course of excluding potential subjects, cohorts may be selected that are unusual and not representative of most patients with the condition.

MATCHING

Patients can be matched as they enter a study so that for each patient in one group there are one or more patients in the comparison group with the same characteristics except for the factor of interest. Often patients are matched for age and sex, because these factors are strongly related to the prognosis of many diseases. But matching for other factors may be called for as well, such as stage or severity of disease, rate of progression, and prior treatments. An example of matching in a cohort study of sickle-cell trait was presented in the discussion of observational studies in Chapter 5.

Although matching is commonly used and can be very useful, it controls for bias only for those factors involved in the match. Also, it is usually not possible to match for more than a few factors, because of practical difficulties in finding patients who meet all the matching criteria. Moreover, if categories for matching are relatively crude, there may be room for substantial differences between matched groups. For example, if a study of risk for Down's syndrome were conducted in which there was matching for maternal age within 10 years, there could be a nearly 10-fold difference in frequency related to age if most of the women in one group were 30 and most in the other 39. Also, once one restricts or matches on a variable, its effects on outcomes can no longer be evaluated in the study.

STRATIFICATION

After data are collected, they can be analyzed and results presented according to subgroups of patients, or *strata*, of similar characteristics.

> *Example* Let us suppose we want to compare the operative mortality rates for coronary bypass surgery at hospitals A and B. Overall, hospital A noted 48 deaths in 1200 bypass operations (4%), and hospital B experienced 64 deaths in 2400 operations (2.6%).
>
> The crude rates suggest that hospital B is superior. Or do they? Perhaps patients in the two hospitals were not otherwise of comparable prognosis. On the basis of age, myocardial function, extent of occlusive disease, and other characteristics, the patients can be divided into subgroups based on preoperative risk (Table 6.3); then the operative mortality rates within each category or stratum of risk can be compared.
>
> Table 6.3 shows that when patients are divided by preoperative risk, the operative mortality rates in each risk stratum are identical in two hospitals: 6% in high-risk patients, 4% in medium-risk patients, and 0.67% in low-risk patients. The obvious source of the misleading impression created by

Table 6.3
Example of Stratification: Hypothetical Death Rates after Coronary Bypass Surgery in Two Hospitals, Stratified by Preoperative Risk

Preoperative Risk	Hospital A			Hospital B		
	Patients	Deaths	Rate (%)	Patients	Deaths	Rate (%)
High	500	30	6	400	24	6
Medium	400	16	4	800	32	4
Low	300	2	0.67	1200	8	0.67
Total	1200	48	4	2400	64	2.6

examining only the crude rates is the important differences in the risk characteristics of the patients treated at the two hospitals: 42% of hospital A's
patients and only 17% of hospital B's patients were high risk.

Stratification is one of the most common and most revealing ways of
examining for bias.

STANDARDIZATION

Two rates can be compared without bias if they are adjusted so as to
equalize the weight given to another factor that could be related to outcome. This process, called *standardization* (or *adjustment*), shows what the
overall rate would be if strata-specific rates were applied to a population
made up of similar proportions of people in each stratum. In the previous
example, the mortality rate of 6% for high-risk patients receives a weight
of 500/1200 in hospital A and a much lower weight of 400/2400 in hospital
B, and so on, such that the crude rate for hospital A = (500/1200 × 0.06)
+ (400/1200 × 0.04) + (300/1200 − 0.0067) = 0.04 and the crude rate for
hospital B equals (400/2400 × 0.06) + (800/2400 × 0.04) + (1200/2400 ×
0. 0067) = 0.026.

If equal weights are used, let us say 1/3 (but they could be based on
one or the other hospital or any reference population), then the standardized rate for hospital A = (1/3 × 0.06) + (1/3 × 0.04) + (1/3 × 0.0067)
= 0.036, which is exactly the same as the standardized rate for hospital B.
The consequence of giving equal weight to strata in each group is to remove
totally the apparent excess risk of hospital A.

The difference between the crude operative mortality rates in the two
hospitals results from the bias introduced by the differences in patients'
preoperative risk. We are only interested in differences attributable to the
hospitals and their surgeons, not to the patients per se. The difference in
the crude mortality rates is confounded by the differences in patients,
whereas standardized mortality rates equalize the weight of patients' preoperative risk in the two hospitals. Standardization is found much more

commonly in studies of risk (in which rates are frequently standardized for age, sex, and/or race) than in studies of prognosis. In contrast to stratification (which is often used in prognosis studies), standardization removes the effect of the extraneous factor. With stratification, the effect can still be examined, even if controlled for. Thus, with standardization, we found that patients had similar prognoses in hospitals A and B. With stratification, we also learned the mortality rates among patients in different risk strata.

MULTIVARIABLE ADJUSTMENT

In most clinical situations, many factors act together to produce effects. The associations among these variables are complex. They may be related to each other as well as to the outcome of interest, the effect of one might be modified by the presence of others, and the joint effects of two or more might be greater than the sum of their individual effects.

Multivariable analysis is a method for simultaneously considering the effects of many variables (Chapter 9). It is used to adjust (control) simultaneously for the effects of many variables to determine the independent effects of one. Also, the method can select from a large set of variables a smaller subset that independently and significantly contributes to the overall variation in outcome and can arrange variables in order of the strength of their contribution. *Cox's proportional hazard analysis* is a type of multivariable analysis used when the outcome is the time to an event (as in survival analyses).

Multivariable analysis is the only feasible way to deal with many variables at one time during the analysis phase of a study. (Randomization also controls for multiple variables, but during the design and conduct phases of a study.) Simpler methods, such as stratification or matching, can only consider a few variables at a time and then only by sacrificing statistical power.

SENSITIVITY ANALYSIS

When data on important prognostic factors are not available, it is possible to estimate the potential effects on the study by assuming various degrees of maldistribution of the factors between the groups being compared and seeing how that would affect the results. The general term for this process is *sensitivity analysis*. The best case/worst case analysis, described earlier in this chapter, is a special type of sensitivity analysis in which one compares results assuming the best and worst possible maldistribution of a prognostic variable.[2]

Assuming the worst is a particularly stringent test of how a factor might affect the conclusions of a study. A less conservative approach is to assume that the factor is distributed between the groups in an unlikely way.

---

[2] Sensitivity analysis can also be used to assess the potential effects of inaccuracies in the data used in decision analysis as discussed in Chapter 4.

Example A study of treatment for mild diabetes found that patients given the sulfonylurea tolbutamide experienced a greater risk of dying from cardiovascular disease than those given insulin or diet alone. The results were criticized because data on smoking—known to be associated with cardiovascular death—were not collected and not taken into account in the analysis. It was suggested that if cigarette smokers were unequally distributed among the groups, such that there were more smokers among those receiving tolbutamide than in the other groups, then the difference in death rates might be related to smoking, not tolbutamide. However, Cornfield (10) pointed out that even if cigarette smokers in the tolbutamide group exceeded those in the control group by 20%, a situation that would have been extremely unlikely by chance (1/50,000), an increased risk in the tolbutamide group would have persisted. Thus bias in the distribution of smokers was unlikely to have accounted for the observed differences.

OVERALL STRATEGY

Except for randomization, all ways of dealing with extraneous differences between groups have a limitation: They are effective against only those factors that are singled out for consideration. They do not deal with prognostic factors that are not known at the time of the study or are known but not taken into account.

Ordinarily, one does not rely on only one or another method of controlling for bias; one uses several methods together, layered one on another. Thus in a study of whether the presence of ventricular premature contractions decreases survival in the years following acute myocardial infarction, one might (*a*) restrict the study to patients who are not very old or young and do not have unusual causes (e.g., mycotic aneurysm) for their infarction; (*b*) match for age, a factor strongly related to prognosis but extraneous to the main question; (*c*) examine the results separately for strata of differing clinical severity (e.g., the presence or absence of congestive heart failure or other diseases, such as chronic obstructive pulmonary disease); and (*d*) using multivariable analysis, adjust the crude results for the effects of all the variables other than the arrhythmia, taken together, that might be related to prognosis.

Generalizability and Sampling Bias

Published accounts of disease prognosis that are based on experience in special centers can paint a misleading picture of prognosis in less selected patients. This is so even if a study is well done, biases are carefully controlled for, and the reported prognosis for a medical condition is correct for the particular sample of patients. Because of the sample of patients used, it may be that the study findings are not generalizable to most other patients with the condition, or to your patient.

Sometimes, patients in randomized controlled trials who are assigned to the control group are studied to better determine the usual clinical course of a disease. But such patients may not be representative of most patients because volunteers for studies tend to do better than patients who do not volunteer. For example, in a large Canadian study of breast cancer screening among women in their 40s, 90% of women who were in the control group and had invasive breast cancer were alive 7 years later, and the number of deaths from breast cancer were lower than for Canadian women generally (11).

Summary

Prognosis is a description of the course of disease from its onset. Compared to risk, prognostic events are relatively frequent and often can be estimated by personal clinical experience. However, cases of disease ordinarily seen in medical centers and reported in the medical literature are often biased samples of all cases and tend to overestimate severity.

Prognosis is best described by the probability of having experienced an outcome event at any time in the course of disease. In principle, this can be done by observing a cohort of patients until all who will experience the outcome of interest have done so. However, because this approach is inefficient, another method—called survival, or time-to-event analysis— is often used. The onset of events over time is estimated by accumulating the rates for all patients at risk during the preceding time intervals.

As for any observations on cohorts, studies comparing prognosis in different groups of patients can be biased if differences arise because of the way cohorts are assembled, if patients do not remain in their initial groups, and if outcome events are not assessed equally. A variety of strategies are available to deal with such differences as might arise, so as to allow fair (unbiased) comparisons. These include restriction, matching, stratification, standardization, multivariable analysis, and sensitivity analysis. One or more of these strategies should be found whenever comparisons are made.

REFERENCES

1. Laupacis A. Changes in quality of life and functional capacity in hemodialysis patients treated with recombinant human erythropoietin. The Canadian Erythropoietin Study Group. Semin Nephrol 1990;2(Suppl 1)1:11–19.
2. Gelber RD et al. Quality-of-life evaluation in a clinical trial of zidovidine therapy in patients with mildly symptomatic HIV infection. Ann Intern Med 1992;116:961–966.
3. Justice AC, Feinstein AR, Wells CK. A new prognostic staging system for the acquired immunodeficiency syndrome. N Eng J Med 1989;320:1388–1393.
4. Wolmark N et al. The prognostic significance of preoperative carcinoembryonic antigen levels in colorectal cancer. Results from the NSABP clinical trials. Ann Surg 1984;199:375–382.
5. Bridges AJ, Conley C, Wang G, Burns DE, Vasey FB. A clinical and immunologic evaluation of women with silicone breast implants and symptoms of rheumatic disease. Ann Intern Med 1993;118:929–936.
6. Gabriel SE, O'Fallon WM, Kurland LT, Beard CM, Woods JE, Melton LJ III. Risk of

connective-tissue diseases and other disorders after breast implantation. N Engl J Med 1994;330:1697–1702.

7. Thompson KS, Fletcher SW, O'Malley MS, Buckwalter JA. Long-term outcomes of morbidly obese patients treated with gastrogastrostomy. J Gen Intern Med 1986;1:85–99.

8. Paffenbarger RS, Hyde RT, Wing AL, Lee IM, Jung DL, Kampert JB. The association of changes in physical-activity level and other lifestyle characteristics with mortality among men. N Eng J Med 1993;328:538–545.

9. Chambers BR, Norris JW. Outcome in patients with asymptomatic neck bruits. N Engl J Med 1986;315:860–865.

10. Cornfield J. The University Group Diabetes Program. A further statistical analysis of the mortality findings. JAMA 1971;217:1676–1687.

11. Miller AB, Baines CJ, Teress Te, Wall C. Canadian National Breast Screening Study. 1. Breast cancer detection and death rates among women aged 40 to 49 years. Can Med Assoc J 1992:147:1459–1476.

SUGGESTED READINGS

Colton T. Statistics in medicine. Boston: Little, Brown, 1975, pp. 237–250.

Concato J, Feinstein AR, Holford TR. The risk of determining risk with multivariable models. Ann Intern Med 1993;118:201–210.

Feinstein AR, Sosin DM, Wells CK. The Will Rogers phenomenon—stage migration and new diagnostic techniques as a source of misleading statistics for survival in cancer. N Engl J Med 1985;312:1604–1608.

Guyatt GH, Feeny DH, Patrick DL. Measuring health-related quality of life. Ann Intern Med 1993;118:622–629.

Horwitz RI. The experimental paradigm and observational studies of cause-effect relationships in clinical medicine. J Chron Dis 1987;40:91–99.

Laupacis A, Wells G, Richardson S, Tugwell P. Users' guides to the medical literature. V. How to use an article about prognosis. JAMA 1994;272:234–237.

Peto R et al. Design and analysis of randomized clinical trials requiring prolonged observation of each patient. II. Analysis and examples. Br J Cancer 1977;35:1–39.

Wasson JH, Sox HC, Neff RK, Goldman L. Clinical prediction rules: applications and methodological standards. N Engl J Med 1985;313:793–799.

Weiss NS: Clinical epidemiology: the study of the outcomes of illness. New York: Oxford University Press, 1986.

7

TREATMENT

Once the nature of a patient's illness has been established and its expected course predicted, the next question is, What can be done about it? Is there a treatment that improves the outcome of disease? This chapter describes the evidence used to decide whether a well-intentioned treatment is effective.

Ideas and Evidence

The discovery of new treatments requires both rich sources of promising possibilities and ways of establishing that the treatments are in fact useful.

IDEAS

Ideas (hypotheses) about what might be useful treatment arise from virtually any activity within medicine. Some therapeutic hypotheses are suggested by the mechanisms of disease at the cellular or molecular level. Drugs against antibiotic resistant bacteria are developed through knowledge of the mechanism of resistance. Hormone analogues are based on the structure of native hormones. The effectiveness of afterload reduction in congestive heart failure was suggested by studies of the importance of afterload in the pathophysiology of heart failure.

Other hypotheses about treatments have come from astute observations by clinicians. Two examples are the discovery that patients with Parkinson's disease who are given amantadine to prevent influenza show improvement in their neurologic status and the reports that colchicine, given for gout, reduces the frequency of attacks of familial Mediterranean fever. The value of these treatments was not predicted by an understanding of the mechanism of these diseases, and the ways in which these drugs work are not yet understood. Similarly, folk remedies from throughout the world, bolstered by centuries of experience but few scientific studies, are potentially useful treatments.

Other ideas come from trial and error. Some anticancer drugs have been found by methodically screening huge numbers of substances for activity.

Ideas about treatment, but more often prevention, also come from epidemiologic studies of populations. Burkitt observed that colonic diseases are less frequent in African countries, where diet is high in fiber, than in developed countries, where intake of dietary fiber is low. This observation has led to efforts to prevent bowel diseases—irritable bowel syndrome, diverticulitis, appendicitis, and colorectal cancer—with high-fiber diets. Comparisons across countries have also suggested the value of red wine to prevent heart disease and fluoride to prevent dental caries.

TESTING IDEAS

Some treatment effects are so prompt and powerful that their value is self-evident even without formal testing. Clinicians do not have reservations about the value of penicillin for pneumonia, surgery for appendicitis, or colchicine for gout. Clinical experience has been sufficient.

Usually, however, the effects of treatment are considerably less dramatic. It is then necessary to put ideas about treatments to a formal test, through clinical research, because a variety of conditions—coincidence, faulty comparisons, spontaneous changes in the course of disease, wishful thinking—can obscure the true relationship between treatment and effect.

Sometimes knowledge of mechanisms of disease, based on work with laboratory models or physiologic studies in humans, has become so extensive that it is tempting to predict effects in humans without formal testing. However, relying solely on our current understanding of mechanisms, without testing ideas on intact humans, can lead to unpleasant surprises because the mechanisms are only partly understood.

> *Example* Many strokes are caused by cerebral infarction in the area distal to an obstructed segment of the internal carotid artery. It should be possible to prevent the manifestations of disease in people with these lesions by bypassing the diseased segment so that blood can flow to the threatened area normally. It is technically feasible to anastamose the superficial temporal artery to the internal carotid distal to an obstruction. Because its value seemed self-evident on physiologic grounds and because of the documented success of an analogous procedure, coronary artery bypass, the surgery became widely used.
>
> The EC/IC Bypass Study Group (1) conducted a randomized controlled trial of temporal artery bypass surgery. Patients with cerebral ischemia and an obstructed internal carotid artery were randomly allocated to surgical versus medical treatment. The operation was a technical success; 96% of anastomoses were patent just after surgery. Yet, the surgery did not help the patients. Mortality and stroke rates after 5 years were nearly identical in the surgically and medically treated patients, but deaths occurred earlier in the surgically treated patients.
>
> This study illustrates how treatments that make good sense, based on what we know about the mechanisms of disease, may be found ineffective in human terms when put to a rigorous test. Of course, it is not always the case that ideas are debunked; the value of carotid endarterectomy, suggested on similar grounds, has been confirmed (2).

Therefore, it is almost always necessary to test therapeutic hypotheses by means of clinical research, in which data are collected on the clinical course of treated and untreated patients. As one author (3) put it, treatments should be given "not because they ought to work, but because they do work."

Studies of Treatment Effects

Treatment is usually considered to be what physicians prescribe for patients with established disease: surgery, drugs, diet and exercise. But there are a great many other ways of intervening to improve health. Among these are efforts to prevent disease in individual patients (counseling and early detection with treatment, discussed in Chapter 8), intervention on communities and changes in the organization and financing of health care. Regardless of the nature of a well-intentioned intervention, the principles by which it is judged superior to its alternatives are the same.

There are two general ways to establish the effects of treatment: observational and experimental studies. They differ in their scientific strength and feasibility.

Observational studies of treatment are a special case of studies of prognosis in general, where the prognostic factor of interest is a therapeutic intervention. What has been said about cohort studies (Chapters 5 and 6) applies to observational studies of treatment as well. The main advantage of these studies is that they are feasible. The main drawback is the likelihood that there are systematic differences in treatment groups other than the treatment itself, which lead to misleading conclusions about the effects of treatment.

Clinical trials are a special kind of cohort study in which the conditions of study—selection of treatment groups, nature of interventions, management during follow-up, and measurement of outcomes—are specified by the investigator for the purpose of making unbiased comparisons. Clinical trials are more highly controlled and managed than are cohort studies. The investigators are conducting an experiment, analogous to those done in the laboratory. They have taken it upon themselves (with their patients' permission) to isolate for study the unique contribution of one factor by holding constant, as much as possible, all other determinants of the outcome. Hence, other names for clinical trials are *experimental* and *intervention* studies.

Randomized controlled trials are the standard of excellence for scientific studies of the effects of treatment. We will consider them in detail first, then consider alternative ways of answering the same question.

Randomized Controlled Trials

The structure of a clinical trial is shown in Figure 7.1. The patients to be studied are first selected from a larger number of patients with the condition of interest. They are then divided, using randomization, into two

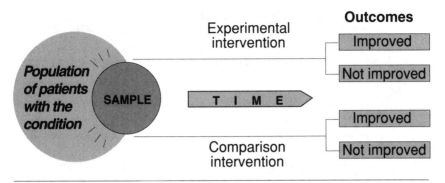

Figure 7.1. The structure of a clinical trial.

groups of comparable prognosis. One group, called the *experimental* or treated group, is exposed to an intervention that is believed to be helpful. The other group, called a *control* or comparison group, is treated the same in all ways except that its members are not exposed to the intervention. The clinical course of both groups is then observed and any differences in outcome are attributed to the intervention.

The main reason for structuring clinical trials in this way is to avoid bias (systematic error) when comparing the respective value of the two or more kinds of treatments. The validity of clinical trials depends on how well they result in an equal distribution of all determinants of prognosis, other than the one being tested, in treated and control patients.

In the following discussion, we will describe the design and interpretation of clinical trials in detail, with reference to Figure 7.2.

SAMPLING

The kinds of patients that are included in a trial determine the extent to which conclusions can be generalized to other patients. Of the many reasons why patients with the condition of interest may not be part of a trial, three account for most of the losses: They do not meet specific entry criteria, they refuse to participate, or they do not cooperate with the conduct of the trial.

The first, entry criteria, is intended to restrict the heterogeneity of patients in the trial. Common exclusion criteria are atypical disease, the presence of other diseases, an unusually poor prognosis (which may cause patients to drop out of the assigned treatment group), and evidence of unreliability. Patients with contraindications to one of the treatments are also excluded, for obvious reasons. As heterogeneity is restricted in this way, the internal validity of the study is improved; there is less opportunity for differences in outcome that are not related to treatment itself. Also, generalizing the results is more precise because one knows exactly to whom

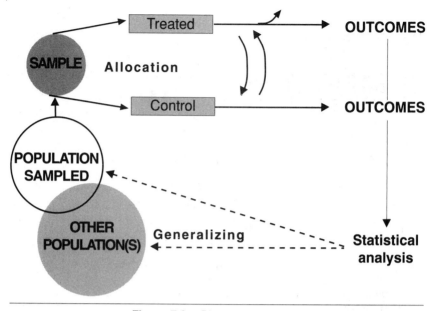

Figure 7.2.   Bias in clinical trials.

the results apply. But exclusions come at the price of diminished scope of generalizability, because characteristics that exclude patients occur commonly among those ordinarily seen in clinical practice, limiting generalizability to these patients, the very ones for whom the information is needed.

Second, patients can refuse to participate in a trial. They may not want a particular type of treatment or to have their medical care decided by a flip of a coin or by someone other than their own physician. Patients who refuse to participate are usually systematically different—in socioeconomic class, severity of disease, other health-related problems, and other ways—from those who agree to enter the trial.

Third, patients who are found to be unreliable during the early stages of the trial are excluded. This avoids wasted effort and the reduction in internal validity that would occur if patients moved in and out of treatment groups or out of the trial altogether.

For these reasons, patients in clinical trials are usually a highly selected, biased sample of all patients with the condition of interest (Fig. 7.3). Because of the high degree of selection in trials, it often requires considerable faith to generalize the results of clinical trials to ordinary practice settings.

INTERVENTION

The intervention itself can be described in relation to three general characteristics: generalizability, complexity, and strength.

First, Is the intervention in question one that is likely to be implemented

Percent of Patients

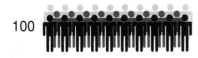

100   **Population Sampled**

Patients with noninsulin-
dependent diabetes mellitus in one
hospital

Inclusion Criteria

Age >40 years
Diabetes diagnosed after 30 years old
Require medication for hyperglycemia
Plan to remain in practice >2 years
Other illness, disability, etc.

24   **Eligible**

Uncooperative

Refused to participate
Did not keep appointments

13   **Randomized**

Dropped Out

Death
Change of residence
Illness, etc.

12   **Completed Study**

Figure 7.3. Sampling for a clinical trial. A study of the effectiveness of a program to reduce lower extremity problems in patients with diabetes. (Data from Litzelman DK, Slemenda CW, Langfeld CD, Hays LM, Welch MA, Bild DE, Ford ES, Vinicor F. Reduction in lower extremity clinical abnormalities in patients with non-insulin dependent diabetes mellitus. A randomized controlled trial. Ann Intern Med 1993;119: 36–41.)

in usual clinical practice? In an effort to standardize therapy so it can be easily described and reproduced in other settings, some investigators end up studying treatments that are so unlike those in usual practice that the results of the trial are not useful.

Second, single, highly specific interventions make for tidy science, because they can be described precisely and applied in a reproducible way. However, clinicians regularly make choices among alternative treatments that involve many elements. Multifaceted interventions are amenable to careful evaluation as long as their essence can be communicated and reproduced in other settings.

> *Example* Falls are a major problem in the elderly, have a variety of causes, and tend to recur. Rubenstein et al. (4) studied the effects of a program to prevent falls in the elderly. Elderly people in a long-term residential care facility were randomized after a fall to a special program or to usual care. The program included a detailed examination, laboratory tests, and environmental assessment; therapeutic recommendations were given to the patient's primary physician. Over the next 2 years, the intervention group had fewer falls, 26% fewer hospitalizations, and a 52% reduction in hospital days compared with controls.

Third, Is the intervention in question sufficiently different from alternative managements that it is reasonable to expect that outcome will be affected? Some diseases can be reversed by treating a single, dominant cause, e.g., treating hyperthyroidism with radioisotope ablation or surgery. But most diseases arise from a combination of factors acting in concert. Interventions that change only one of them, and only a small amount, cannot be expected to show strong treatment effects. If the conclusion of a trial evaluating such interventions is that a new treatment is not effective, it should come as no surprise.

COMPARISON GROUPS

The value of a treatment can only be judged by comparing the results of the treatment to those of some alternative course of action. The question is not whether a point of comparison is used, but how appropriate it is. Results among patients receiving an experimental treatment can be measured against one or more of several kinds of comparison groups.

No Intervention

Do patients receiving the experimental treatment end up better than those receiving nothing at all? Comparing treatment with no treatment measures the total effects of health care, both specific and nonspecific.

Observation

Do treated patients do better than other patients who are simply observed? A great deal of special attention is directed toward patients in clinical trials, and they are well aware of it. People have a tendency to change their behavior because they are the target of special interest and attention in a study, regardless of the specific nature of the intervention they might be receiving, a phenomenon called the *Hawthorne effect*. The reasons for this changed behavior are not clear. Patients are anxious to please their doctors and make them feel successful. Also, patients who volunteer for trials want to do their part to see that "good" results are obtained. Thus comparison of treatment with simple observation measures treatment effect over and above the Hawthorne effect.

Placebo Treatment

Do treated patients do better than similar patients given a *placebo*, an intervention that is intended to be indistinguishable from the active treatment—in physical appearance, color, taste, and smell—but does not have a specific, known mechanism of action? Sugar pills and saline injections are examples of placebos. It has been shown that placebos, given with conviction, relieve severe, unpleasant symptoms, such as postoperative pain, nausea, or itching, of about one-third of patients, a phenomenon called the *placebo effect*.

> *Example* Patients with chronic severe itching were entered in a trial of antipruritic drugs. During each of 3 weeks, 46 patients received in random order either cyproheptadine HCl, trimeprazine tartrate, or placebo. There was a 1-week rest period, randomly introduced into the sequence, in which no pills were given. Results were assessed without knowledge of medication and expressed as "itching scores"; the higher the score, the worse the itching. Itching scores for the various treatments were cyproheptadine HCl, 28; trimeprazine tartrate, 35; placebo, 30; and no treatment, 50. The two active drugs and placebo were all similarly effective and all gave much better results than no treatment (5).

Placebo effects have different meaning for researchers and clinicians. Researchers are more likely to be interested in establishing specific effects—ones that are consistent with current theories about the causes of disease. They consider the placebo effect the baseline against which to measure specific effects. Clinicians, on the other hand, should welcome the placebo effect and attempt to maximize it or any other way of helping patients.

Many clinical interventions have both specific and nonspecific effects (Fig. 7.4). What is important to clinicians and their patients is the total effect of the intervention beyond what would have otherwise occurred in the course of disease without treatment. However, it is also useful to know what part of the total effect is specific and what is nonspecific so as to avoid dangerous, uncomfortable, or costly interventions when relatively little of their effect can be attributed to their specific actions.

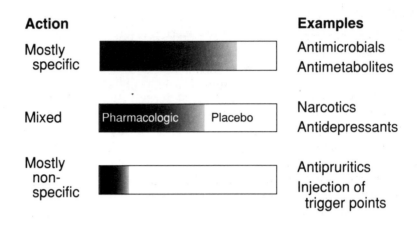

Figure 7.4. The effects of most drugs are partly attributable to the placebo effect. (Redrawn from Fletcher RH. The clinical importance of placebo effects. Fam Med Rev 1983;1:40–48.)

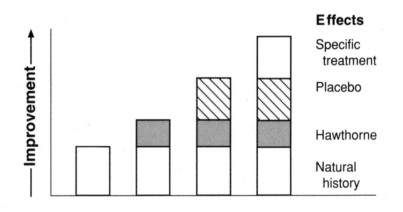

Figure 7.5. Total effects of treatment are the sum of spontaneous improvement, nonspecific responses, and the effects of specific treatments.

Usual Treatment

Do patients given the experimental treatment do better than those receiving usual treatment? This is the only meaningful (and ethical) question if the usual treatment is already known to be efficacious.

The cumulative effects of these various reasons for improvement in treated patients are diagrammed in Figure 7.5.

ALLOCATING TREATMENT

To study the effects of a clinical intervention free of other effects, the best way to allocate patients to treatment groups is by means of *randomization*. Patients are given either the experimental or the control treatment by one of a variety of disciplined procedures—analogous to flipping a coin— whereby each patient has an equal (or at least known) chance of being assigned to any one of the treatment groups.

Random allocation of patients is preferable to other methods of allocation, because randomization assigns patients to groups without bias. That is, patients in one group are, on the average, as likely to possess a given characteristic as patients in another. Only with randomization is this so for all factors related to prognosis, whether or not they are known before the study takes place.

In the long run, with a large number of patients in the trial, randomization usually works as described above. However, random allocation does not guarantee that the groups will be similar. Although the process of random allocation is unbiased, the results may not be. Dissimilarities between groups can arise by chance alone, particularly when the number of patients randomized is small. To assess whether this kind of "bad luck" has occurred, authors of randomized controlled trials often present a table comparing the frequency of a variety of characteristics in the treated and control groups, especially those known to be related to outcome. It is reassuring to see that important characteristics have, in fact, fallen out nearly equally in the groups being compared. If they have not, it is possible to see what the differences are and attempt to control them in the analysis (see Chapter 6).

Some investigators believe it is best to make sure, before randomization, that at least some of the characteristics known to be strongly associated with outcome appear equally in treated and control groups, to reduce the risk of bad luck. They suggest that patients first be gathered into groups (strata) of similar prognosis and then randomized separately within each stratum—a process called *stratified randomization*. The groups are then bound to be comparable, at least for the characteristics that were used to create the strata. Others argue that whatever differences arise by bad luck are unlikely to be large and can be dealt with mathematically after the data are collected.

DIFFERENCES ARISING AFTER RANDOMIZATION

Not all patients in a clinical trial participate as originally planned. Some are found not to have the disease they were thought to have when they entered the trial. Others drop out, do not take their medications, are taken out of the study because of side effects or other illnesses, or somehow obtain the other study treatment or treatments that are not part of the study at all. The result is comparison of treatment groups that might have been comparable just after randomization but have become less so by the time outcomes are counted.

Patients Do Not Have the Disease

It may be necessary to decide which treatment to give (in a clinical trial or in practice) before it is certain the patient actually has the disease for which the treatment is designed.

> *Example* To study whether a monoclonal antibody against endotoxin improves survival from sepsis, 543 patients with sepsis and suspected Gram-negative infection were randomized to receive antiendotoxin or placebo (6). In the subgroup of patients who actually had Gram-negative bacteremia, death rate was reduced from 49 to 30%, a large difference that was well beyond what could be accounted for by chance. However, only 200 patients (37%) had Gram-negative bacteremia, confirmed by blood culture. There is no known reason why the other 63% would be helped by the drug. For all patients with sepsis (some of whom had bacteremia and others did not) mortality rate was 43% in the placebo group and 39% in the group receiving antiendotoxin, a small difference that was not beyond that expected by chance alone.
>
> Thus, from this trial, there was evidence that the drug was effective against Gram-negative bacteremia, but not for sepsis. Both are important questions: the former for researchers, who are interested in the biologic effect of antiendotoxin in bacteremia, and the latter for clinicians, who needed to know the clinical effects of their decision to give the drug to patients with sepsis—a decision that must be made before it is known whether or not bacteremia is actually present.

When patients suspected of having the specific disease in question later turn out not to have it, there is a price to pay. Studying additional patients who could not benefit from the specific action of the treatment decreases the efficiency of the trial; more patients must be studied to see the effect. Looked at another way, because patients experiencing the specific effect are mixed with others who cannot, the effect size is reduced relative to a trial including only patients with the disease. This decreases the chances, for a given number of patients in the trial, that an effect will be found (see Chapter 9). However, this kind of trial has the important advantage of providing information on the consequences of a decision as the clinician encounters it (see "Management and Explanatory Trials," later in this chapter).

Compliance

Compliance is the extent to which patients follow medical advice. Some prefer the term *adherence,* because it connotes a less subservient relationship between patient and doctor. Compliance is another characteristic of patients that can arise after randomization. Although noncompliance suggests a kind of willful neglect of good advice, in medicine other factors also contribute. Patients may misunderstand which drugs and doses are intended, run out of prescription medications, confuse various prepara-tions of the same drug, or have no money or insurance to pay for drugs. Taken together, these may limit the usefulness of treatments that have been shown to work under specially favorable conditions.

Compliance is particularly important in medical care outside the hospi-tal. In the hospital, many factors act to constrain patients' personal behavior and render them compliant. Hospitalized patients are generally sicker and more frightened. They are in strange surroundings, dependent on the skill and attention of the staff for everything—even their life. What is more, doctors, nurses, and pharmacists have developed a well-organized system for ensuring that patients receive what is ordered for them. As a result, clinical experience and a medical literature developed on the wards may underestimate the importance of compliance outside the hospital, where most patients and doctors are and where doing what clinicians advise is more difficult.

Comparing responses among compliant and noncompliant patients in a randomized trial can be misleading.

> *Example* During a large study of the effects of several lipid-lowering drugs on coronary heart disease, 1103 men were given clofibrate and 2789 men were given placebo. The 5-year mortality rate was 20.0% for the clofi-brate group and 20.9% for the placebo group, indicating that the drug was not effective.
>
> It was recognized that not all patients took their medications. Was clofi-brate effective among patients who actually took the drug? The answer ap-peared to be yes. Among patients given clofibrate, 5-year mortality for pa-tients taking most of their prescribed drug was 15.0%, compared with 24.6% for the less cooperative patients ($p < 10^{-5}$). However, taking the prescribed drug was also related to lower mortality rates among patients prescribed placebo. For them, 5-year mortality was 15.1% for patients taking most of their placebo medication and 28.3 for patients who did not ($p < 10^{-15}$). Thus there was an association between drug taking and prognosis that was not related to the active drug itself.
>
> The authors (7) cautioned against evaluating treatment effects in sub-groups determined by patient responses to the treatment protocol after randomization.

Cointerventions

After randomization, patients may receive a variety of interventions other than the ones being studied. If these occur unequally in the two groups and affect outcomes, they can introduce systematic differences (bias) between the groups compared.

> *Example* The care of AIDS is emotional, in part because it affects young adults and is universally fatal within a few years of the onset of symptoms. Efforts to study the effectiveness of treatment have been hindered by disrup-tion of the usual procedures of randomized trials, as patients try to maximize their chances of survival. Patients in randomized trials sometimes exchange

the drugs being studied in the trial (researchers call the exchange of treatment regimens among study participants "contamination") or obtain drugs that are not part of the trial through "drug clubs." Information about this behavior is usually not shared with the researchers and so cannot be accounted for in the study. The result is to bias the study toward observing no effect, since the contrast between the treatment of the "treated" group and the comparison group is diminished.

Comparing Responders with Nonresponders

In some clinical trials, particularly those about cancer, the outcomes of patients who initially improve after treatment (responders) are compared with outcomes in those who do not (nonresponders). The implication is that one can learn something about the efficacy of treatment in this way.

This approach is scientifically unsound and often misleading, because response and nonresponse might be associated with many characteristics related to the ultimate outcome: stage of disease, rate of progression, compliance, dose and side effects of drugs, and the presence of other diseases. If no patient actually improved because of the treatment, and patients were destined to follow various clinical courses for other reasons, then some (the ones who happened to be doing well) would be called "responders" and others (the ones having a bad course) would be considered "nonresponders." Responders would, of course, have a better outcome whether or not they received the experimental treatment.

BLINDING

Participants in a trial may change their behavior in a systematic way (i.e., be biased) if they are aware of which patients receive which treatment. One way to minimize this effect is by *blinding,* an attempt to make the various participants in a study unaware of which treatment patients have been offered, so that the knowledge does not cause them to act differently, thereby damaging the internal validity of the study. "Masking" is a more appropriate metaphor, but blinding is the time-honored term.

Blinding can take place at four levels in a clinical trial. First, those responsible for allocating patients to treatment groups should not know which treatment will be assigned next so that the knowledge does not affect their willingness to enter patients in the trial or take them in the order they arrived. Second, patients should be unaware of which treatment they are taking; they are thereby less likely to change their compliance or their reporting of symptoms because of this information. Third, physicians who take care of patients in the study should not know which treatment each patient has been given; then they will not, perhaps unconsciously, manage them differently. Finally, if the researchers who assess outcomes cannot distinguish treatment groups, that knowledge cannot affect their measurements.

The terms *single-blind* (patients) and *double-blind* (patients and researchers) are sometimes used, but their meaning is ambiguous. It is better simply to describe what was done. A trial in which there is no attempt at blinding is called *open* or *open label.*

When blinding is possible, mainly for studies of drug effects, it is usually accomplished by means of a placebo. However, for many important clinical questions—the effects of surgery, radiotherapy, diet, or the organization of medical care—blinding of patients and managing physicians is not possible.

Even when blinding appears to be possible, it is more often claimed than successful. Physiologic effects, such as lowered pulse rate with beta-blocking drugs, or bone marrow depression with cancer chemotherapy, are regular features of some medications. Symptoms may also be a clue.

> *Example* In the Lipids Research Clinics (8) trial of the primary prevention of cardiovascular disease, a nearly perfect placebo was used. Some people received cholestyramine and others a powder of the same appearance, odor, and taste. However, side effects were substantially more common in the cholestyramine group. At the end of the 1st year of the trial, there were much higher rates in the experimental (cholestyramine) group than the control group for constipation (39 versus 10%), heartburn (27 versus 10%), belching and bloating (27 versus 16%), and nausea (16 versus 8%). Patients might have been prompted by new symptoms to guess which treatment they were getting.

There is also objective evidence that patients and physicians in some blinded trials can guess who received what treatment.

> *Example* A double-blind, randomized trial was conducted to see if propranolol could prevent another myocardial infarction in patients who had already had one (9). At the conclusion of the trial, but before unblinding, patients and clinic personnel were asked to guess the treatment group assignment of each patient. For patients, 79.9% guessed propranolol correctly and 57.2% placebo correctly. Physicians and clinic personnel were similarly accurate. Clinical personnel seemed to be aided in their guessing by observation of heart rate; it was unclear how patients knew.

ASSESSMENT OF OUTCOMES

When the outcome of a trial is measured in unequivocal terms, such as being alive or dead, it is unlikely that patients will be misclassified. On the other hand, when outcomes are decided by the opinion of one of the participants, there is much greater opportunity for bias. For example, although the fact of death is usually clear, the cause of death is often not. Most people die for a combination of reasons or for obscure reasons, allowing some room for judgment in assigning cause of death. This judgment can be influenced by knowledge of what went before, including the treatments that were given. Opportunities for bias are even greater when assessing symptoms such as pain, nausea, or depression. Bias in assessing outcomes is avoided by searching for outcome events equally in all patients, using explicit criteria for when an outcome has occurred, and by blinding.

Short-term, easily measurable "outcomes" may be substituted for clinical ones so as to speed the rate at which trials can be completed and reported. For example, it has been common in clinical trials of treatment of HIV infection to take as the main outcome measures biologic tests that reflect the extent of infection (such as CD4+ counts and p32 antigen) rather than clinical progression of disease (opportunistic infections and death). However, it has been shown that CD4+ counts are an imperfect marker of clinical treatment effect. As discussed in Chapter 1, the practice of substituting biologic outcomes for clinical ones in studies that are to guide patient care is defensible only if the proxy is known to be itself strongly related to the clinical outcome.

There are several options for summarizing the relative effects of two treatments (Table 7.1). It has been suggested that the most clinically relevant expression is *number needed to treat,* the number of patients that must be treated to prevent one outcome event (10). Number needed to treat is the reciprocal of absolute risk reduction.

Perception of the size of a treatment effect, both by patients and clinicians, is influenced by how the effect is reported. In general, effects reported as relative risks seem larger than the same effects described as attributable risks, which in turn seem larger than reports of the number needed to treat (11,12). Also, patients told their probability of survival believe they have a better chance than those told the complement, their probability of dying (13). Thus, to understand and communicate treatment effects, it is necessary to examine the main results of a trial in several ways. It is moot which is the "correct" statistic.

Table 7.1
Summarizing Treatment Effects[a]

Summary Measure[b]	Definition
Relative risk reduction	$\dfrac{\text{Control event rate} - \text{Treated event rate}}{\text{Control event rate}}$
Absolute risk reduction	Control event rate − Treated event rate
Number needed to treat	$\dfrac{1}{\text{Control event rate} - \text{Treated event rate}}$

[a] Laupacis A, Sackett DL, Roberts RS. An assessment of clinically useful measures of the consequences of treatment. New Engl J Med 1988;318:1728–1733.
[b] For continuous data, when there are measurements at baseline and after treatment, analogous measures are based on the mean values for treated and control groups either after treatment or for the difference between baseline and posttreatment values.

MANAGEMENT AND EXPLANATORY TRIALS

The results of a randomized controlled trial can be analyzed and presented in two ways: according to the treatment to which the patients were randomized or to the one they actually received. The correct presentation of results depends on the question being asked.

If the question is which treatment policy is best at the time the decision must be made, then analysis according to the assigned (randomized) group is appropriate—whether or not some patients did not actually receive the treatment they were supposed to receive. Trials analyzed in this way are called *intention to treat* or *management* trials (14). The advantages of this approach are that the question corresponds to the one actually faced by clinicians and the patients compared are really randomized. The disadvantage is that if many patients do not receive the treatment to which they were randomized differences between experimental and control groups will tend to be obscured, increasing the chances of a negative study. Then if the study shows no difference, it is uncertain whether the experimental treatment is truly ineffective or was just not received.

Another question is whether the experimental treatment itself is better? For this question, the proper analysis is according to the treatment each patient actually received, regardless of the treatment to which they were randomized. Trials analyzed in this way are called *explanatory trials* because they emphasize the mechanism by which effects are exerted. The problem with this approach is that unless most patients receive the treatment to which they are assigned the study no longer represents a randomized trial; it is simply a cohort study. Therefore, one must be concerned about dissimilarities between groups, other than the experimental treatment, and must use one or more methods (restriction, matching, stratification, or adjustment) to achieve comparability, just as one would for any nonexperimental study. These two approaches are illustrated in Figure 7.6.

EFFICACY AND EFFECTIVENESS

A trial's results are judged in relation to two broad questions. Can the treatment work under ideal circumstances? Does it work in ordinary settings? The words *efficacy* and *effectiveness* have been applied to these concepts (Fig. 7.7).

The question of whether a treatment can work is one of *efficacy*. An *efficacious* treatment is one that has the desired effects among those who receive it. Efficacy is established by restricting patients in a study to those who will cooperate fully with medical advice.

In contrast, a treatment is *effective* if it does more good than harm in those to whom it is offered. Effectiveness is established by offering a treatment or program to patients and allowing them to accept or reject it as they might ordinarily do. Only a small proportion of clinical trials set out to answer

Intention to Treat Analysis

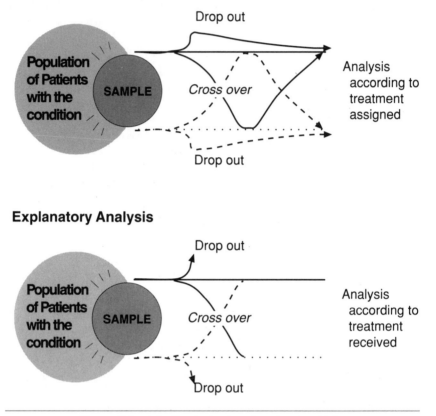

Figure 7.6.   Intention to treat and explanatory trials.

questions of effectiveness. This is in part because of the risk that the result will be inconclusive. If a treatment is found to be ineffective, it could be because of a lack of efficacy, lack of patient acceptance, or both.

Tailoring the Results of Trials to Individual Patients

Clinical trials involve pooling the experience of many patients who are admittedly dissimilar and describing what happens to them on the average. How can we obtain more precise estimates for individual patients? Two ways are to examine subgroups and to study individual patients using rigorous methods similar to those in randomized trials.

SUBGROUPS

The principal result of a clinical trial is a description of the most important outcome in each of the major treatment groups. But it is tempting to examine the results in more detail than the overall conclusions afford.

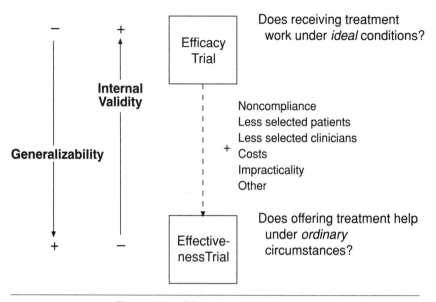

Figure 7.7.   Efficacy and effectiveness.

We look at subgroups of patients with special characteristics or with particular outcomes. In doing so, however, there are some risks of being misled that are not present when examining the principal conclusions alone, and these should be taken into account when interpreting information from subgroups. (Some of the concepts on which this section is based are discussed in Chapter 9.)

One danger in examining subgroups is the increased chance of finding effects in a particular subgroup that are not present, in the long run, in nature. This arises because multiple comparisons lead to a greater chance of a false-positive finding than is estimated by the individual p value for that comparison alone (see Chapter 9). Table 7.2 lists some guidelines for deciding whether a finding in a subgroup is real.

A second danger is of a false-negative conclusion. Examining subgroups in a clinical trial—either certain kinds of patients or specific kinds of outcomes—involves a great reduction in the data available, so it is frequently impossible to come to firm conclusions. Nevertheless, the temptation to look is there, and some tentative information can be gleaned.

> *Example*   The Physicians' Health Study (15) is a randomized controlled trial designed to assess whether daily aspirin prevents mortality from cardiovascular disease in healthy male physicians. Another aspect of the trial is to study the effect of β-carotene on the incidence of cancer. The aspirin part of the study was stopped long before there were enough deaths to determine if aspirin affected mortality, because the physicians had a much lower than

expected death rate. The trial was also stopped because there were fewer myocardial infarctions in the treated than the control group. The authors thought that the effect on myocardial infarction, although not the answer to a main study question at the outset, was real because it was biologically plausible, because it was found in other studies, and because the chance of a false-positive conclusion was estimated to be very small (1/10,000). On the other hand, although the authors observed a small increase in risk of stroke in the treated group, they could not be certain whether this effect was real or not, as there were too few physicians with this end point. Thus, in a study that could not address the main research question, the authors interpreted the validity of findings in subgroups (both positive and negative) in relation to the totality of information that might bear on the validity of these findings.

EFFECTIVENESS IN INDIVIDUAL PATIENTS

A treatment that is effective on the average may not work on an individual patient. The results of valid clinical research provide a good reason to begin treating a patient, but experience with that patient is a better reason to continue therapy. Therefore, when conducting a treatment program it is useful to ask the following series of questions:

- Is the treatment known to be efficacious for any patients?
- Is the treatment known to be effective, on the average, in patients like mine?
- Are the benefits worth the discomforts and risks?
- Is the treatment working in my patient?

By asking these questions, and not simply following the results of trials alone, one can guard against ill-founded choice of treatment or stubborn persistence in the face of poor results.

Table 7.2
Guidelines for Deciding Whether Apparent Differences in Effects within Subgroups Are Real[a]

From the study itself
- Is the magnitude of the observed difference clinically important?
- How likely is the effect to have arisen by chance, taking into account:
  The number of subgroups examined?
  The magnitude of the p value?
- Was a hypothesis that the effect would be observed
  Made before its discovery (or was justification for the effect argued for after it was found)?
  One of a small number of hypotheses?
From other information
- Was the difference suggested by comparisons within rather than between studies?
- Has the effect been observed in other studies?
- Is there indirect evidence that supports the existence of the effect?

[a] Adapted from Oxman AD, Guyatt GH. A consumer's guide to subgroup analysis. Ann Intern Med 1992;116:78–84.

TRIALS OF *N* = 1

Rigorous clinical trials, with proper attention to bias and chance, can be done with individual patients, one at a time (16). The method—called *trials of N* = 1—is an improvement in the more informal process of trial and error that is so common in clinical practice. A patient is given one or another treatment (e.g., active treatment or placebo) in random order, each for a brief period of time, such as a week or two. Patients and physicians are blind to which treatment is given. Outcomes (e.g., a simple preference for a treatment or a symptom score) are assessed after each period and subjected to statistical analysis.

This method is useful when activity of disease is unpredictable, response to treatment is prompt, and there is no carryover effect from period to period. Examples of diseases for which the method can be used include migraine, bronchospasm, fibrositis, and functional bowel disease.

N of 1 trials can be useful for guiding clinical decision making, although for a relatively small proportion of patients. It can also be used to screen interesting clinical hypotheses to select some that are promising enough to be evaluated using a full randomized controlled trial involving many patients.

Alternatives to Randomized Trials

Randomized, controlled, blinded trials are the standard of excellence for comparisons of treatment effects over time. They should be given precedence over other information about treatment effects whenever they are available. However, it is not always possible to rely on clinical trials.

LIMITATIONS OF RANDOMIZED TRIALS

Clinical trials are limited for several reasons. There may not be enough patients with the disease of interest, at one time and place, to carry out a scientifically sound trial. Clinical trials are costly, more than $50–100 million for some large trials. Years pass before results are available, which may be politically unacceptable for severe, emotion-laden diseases such as AIDS.

Sometimes a practice may have become so well established, in the absence of conclusive evidence of its benefit, that it is difficult to convince physicians and potential participants that a trial is needed. It could be argued that if the treatment effect is not really known then the only ethical thing is to do the study (and it is unethical to continue to use treatments of uncertain benefit), but this argument demands a level of analytic reasoning that is uncommon among patients and their physicians. Because of this problem, some physicians have advocated "randomization from the first patient," beginning trials just after a new treatment is introduced. Others argue that it is better to conduct rigorous clinical trials somewhat later, after the best way to deliver the treatment has been worked out, so that a good example of the intervention is tested. In any case, it is generally agreed that if a controlled trial is postponed too long, the opportunity to do it all may be lost.

For these reasons, guidance from clinical trials is not available for many treatment decisions. But the decisions must be made nonetheless. What are the alternatives and how credible are they?

ADVANTAGES AND DISADVANTAGES

Alternatives to randomized trials usually make use of large databases such as those collected for patient care, billing, or administration. Sometime data collected to answer another research question are used. A research question, and a study to answer it, can be devised after the data have been collected so that most of the resources needed for the study go into analyses of the data. This process is called *secondary data analysis,* because answering the research question was not the primary reason for collecting the data.

Using secondary data for research has several advantages, all of them practical. First, if the database includes experience from a large number of patients, as is often the case, then the research question can be answered with a high degree of confidence that the results are not just by chance. It may even be possible to examine subgroups (e.g., elderly women taking estrogens or young men with a first anterior myocardial infarction) with statistical confidence. Most clinical trials are not designed with such an abundance of patients because of the cost; the best trials are sufficient to answer the main research question for all patients in the study but are rarely sufficient to answer questions about subgroups of patients.

Second, these databases are collected in more natural settings than clinical trials. They reflect experience in health care organizations or perhaps entire regions or nations, rather than a highly selected group of experimental subjects. Therefore, the results are more generalizable.

Third, it costs less to use existing data than to collect new data in a clinical trial. Randomized trials cost thousands of dollars per patient to recruit, evaluate, enroll, and follow up each patient, whereas analyses of existing data can be relatively inexpensive.

Finally, by using existing data, it is possible to have an answer to an important question in a relatively short time. Clinical trials often take years from enrollment of the first patient to the end of follow-up. Sometimes clinicians need an answer, however imperfect, sooner because they are making high-stakes decisions on alternative treatments every day.

Balanced against all of these practical advantages are disadvantages. The data are usually not collected and classified with as much care as they would be for a well-run clinical trial. For example, a claims data diagnosis of "hypertension" stands for whatever the responsible physicians believes hypertension is, whereas a research definition of hypertension would specify a level of blood pressure, method, and frequency, perhaps adjusted for age. Some important variables may be missing from the database because they were not important for the database's original purposes, though they are important for the research. Of course, there is also the problem of making unbiased comparisons.

The trade-off between speed and ease, on the one hand, and validity, on the other, will be discussed for each alternative design in the next sections.

COMPARISONS ACROSS TIME AND PLACE

Control patients can be chosen from a time and place different from the experimental patients. For example, we may compare the prognosis of recent patients treated with current medications to experience with past patients who were treated when current medications were not available. Similarly, we may compare the results of surgery in one hospital to results in another, where a different procedure is used. This approach is convenient. The problem is that time and place are almost always strongly related to prognosis. Clinical trials that attempt to make fair comparisons between groups of patients arising in different eras, or in different settings, have a particularly difficult task.

The results of current treatment are sometimes compared with experience with similar patients in the past, called *historical or nonconcurrent controls.* Although it may be done well, this design has many pitfalls. Methods of diagnosis change with time, and with them the average prognosis. It has been shown that new diagnostic technologies have created the impression that the prognosis of treated lung cancer have improved over time when it has not (17). With better ability to detect occult metastases, patients are classified in a worse stage than they would have been earlier, and this "stage migration" has resulted in a better prognosis in each stage than was reported in the past. Supporting treatments (e.g., antibiotics, nutritional supplementation and peptic ulcer prevention) also improve with time, creating a general improvement in prognosis that might not be attributable to the specific treatment given in a later time period.

> *Example*   Sacks et al. (18) reviewed clinical trials of six therapies to see if trials with concurrent controls produced different results than studies of the same treatments with historical controls. They studied 50 randomized trials and 56 studies with historical controls. A total of 79% of trials with historical controls but only 20% of trials with a concurrent, randomized control group found the experimental treatment to be better. Differences between the two kinds of trials occurred mainly because the control patients in the historical trials did worse. Adjustment for prognostic factors, when possible, did not change the results, i.e., the differences were probably because of general improvements in therapy or to selection of less ill patients.

Therefore, if concurrent, randomized controlled trials are taken as a standard of validity it seems that published historical trials are biased in favor of the experimental treatment and that the bias cannot be overcome by adjusting for known prognostic variables.

If historical controls are used, the shorter the period of time between selection of treated and control groups and the less other aspects of medical care have changed during the interval, the safer the comparison. Thus some oncology centers study a succession of chemotherapeutic regimens by comparing results of the newest regimen with those of the immediately preceding one, often given as recently as the previous year. In general, however, choosing *concurrent controls* (i.e., patients treated during the same period of time) is a better way of avoiding bias.

Experience in other settings, using different treatments, can serve as a standard of comparison. However, it is preferable to choose both treated and control patients from the same setting, because a variety of factors— referral patterns, organization and skill of staff, etc.—often result in very different prognoses in different settings, independently of the treatment under study.

> *Example*   The mortality rate for hospitals where coronary bypass surgery was done varied almost threefold across hospitals in central Pennsylvania (Fig. 7.8) (19). The severity of illness, and therefore prognosis, of patients in these hospitals varied too. After taking into account the number of deaths expected, by considering patients' prognostic factors, one hospital had fewer than expected deaths, another the expected number, and a third more than expected. Any fair comparison of treatment effects across these hospitals would have to take into account not only the differences in severity of the patients in these hospitals but also the skills of the surgeons.

UNCONTROLLED TRIALS

Uncontrolled trials describe the course of disease in a single group of patients who have been exposed to the intervention of interest. Another name for this design is a "before-after study." The assumption of this approach is that whatever improvement is observed after treatment is because of treatment. This assumption may be unwarranted for several reasons.

Unpredictable Outcome

When the clinical course of a disease is quite predictable, a separate control group is less important. We know that subacute bacterial endocarditis without antibiotics and rabies without vaccine invariably lead to death, that most patients with hypothyroidism will only get worse without exogenous thyroid hormone, and that bowel infarction will rarely improve without surgery.

However, most therapeutic decisions do not involve conditions with

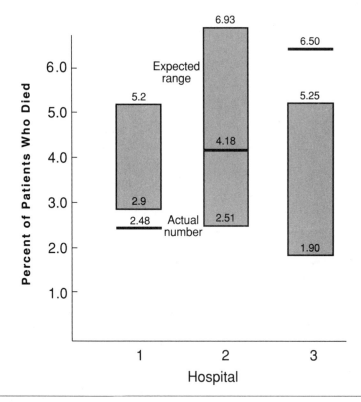

Figure 7.8. Severity of illness and skill of surgeons vary by location. Observed and expected (taking into account case mix) death rate from coronary bypass surgery in three hospitals. (Data from Topol EJ, Califf RM. Scorecard cardiovascular medicine. Its impact and future direction. Ann Intern Med 1994;120:65–70.)

such predictable outcomes. In situations where the clinical course is extremely variable for a given patient and from one patient to another, assessing treatment effects by observing changes in the course of disease after treatment is unreliable.

Many severe diseases that are not self-limited may nevertheless undergo spontaneous remissions in activity that can be misinterpreted as treatment effects. Figure 7.9 shows the clinical course of a patient with systemic lupus erythematosus over a 10-year period, 1955–1964 (20). Although powerful treatments were not given (because none was available during most of these years), the disease passed through dramatic periods of exacerbation, followed by prolonged remissions. Of course, exacerbations, such as those illustrated, are alarming to both patients and doctors, so there is often a feeling that something must be done at these times. If treatment were

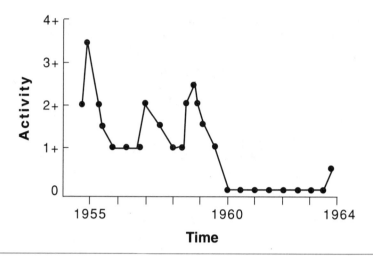

Figure 7.9. The unpredictable course of disease. The natural history of systemic lupus erythematosus in a patient observed before the advent of immunosuppressive drugs. (Redrawn from Ropes M. Systemic lupus erythematosus. Cambridge, MA: Harvard University Press, 1976.)

begun at the peak of activity, improvement would have followed. Without any better comparison than the previous activity of the disease, the treatment would have received credit for the improvement.

Nonspecific Effects

In uncontrolled trials, there is no way of separating Hawthorne and placebo effects from treatment effects. But if there are control patients who receive the same attention as the treated ones and a placebo, then these effects cancel out in the comparison.

Regression to the Mean

Treatments are often tried because a manifestation of disease, e.g., a particularly high blood pressure or fever, is extreme or unusual. In this situation, subsequent measurements are likely to show improvement for purely statistical reasons. As discussed in Chapter 2, patients selected because they represent an extreme high value in a distribution are likely, on the average, to have lower values for later measurements. If those patients are treated after first being found abnormal and the effects of treatment are assessed by subsequent measurements, improvement could be expected even if treatment were ineffective.

Predictable Improvement

The usual course of some diseases is to improve; if so, therapeutic efforts may coincide with improvement but not cause it. For example, patients tend to seek care for many acute, self-limited diseases, such as upper respiratory infections or gastroenteritis, when symptoms are at their worst. They often begin to recover after seeing the doctor because of the natural course of events regardless of what was done.

NONRANDOM ALLOCATION OF TREATMENT

One way to allocate patients to treated and control groups is to have the physicians caring for the patients decide. When this is done, the study has all the advantages and disadvantages of cohort studies.

Studies of treated cohorts take advantage of the fact that therapeutic decisions must be made for sick patients regardless of the quality of existing evidence on the subject. In the absence of a clear-cut consensus favoring one mode of treatment over others, various treatments are often given. As a result, in the course of ordinary patient care large numbers of patients receive various treatments and go on to manifest their effects. If experience with these patients can be captured and properly analyzed, it can be used to guide therapeutic decisions.

Unfortunately, it is often difficult to be sure that observational studies of treatment involve unbiased comparisons. Decisions about treatment are determined by a great many factors—severity of illness, concurrent diseases, local preferences, patient cooperation, etc. Patients receiving the different treatments are likely to differ not only in their treatment but in other ways as well. Efforts to determine the results of treatment alone, free from other factors, are thereby compromised.

Phases of Studies of Treatment

For studies of drugs, it is customary to define three phases of trials, in the order they are undertaken (21). *Phase I trials* are intended to identify a dose range that is well tolerated and safe (at least for high-frequency, severe side effects) and include very small numbers of patients (perhaps a dozen), without a control group. *Phase II trials* provide preliminary information on whether the drug is efficacious and the relationship between dose and efficacy; these trials may be controlled but include too few patients in treatment groups to detect any but the largest treatment effects. They may not be blinded. *Phase III trials* provide definitive evidence of efficacy and the presence of common side effects. They include enough patients—dozens to thousands—to detect clinically important treatment effects and are commonly published in clinical journals and used by regulatory agencies to decide whether to license drugs.

Phase III trials are not large enough to detect differences in the rate—or even the existence—of uncommon side effects. (See discussion of statistical power, Chapter 9.) For this, it is necessary to follow up very large numbers of patients after a drug is in general use, a process called "postmarketing surveillance" or, sometimes, phase IV of drug development.

Summary

Promising ideas about what might be good treatment should be put to a rigorous test before being used as a basis for clinical decisions. The best test is a randomized controlled trial, a special case of a cohort study in which the intervention is allocated randomly and, therefore, without bias. Patients in clinical trials are usually highly selected, reducing generalizability. They are randomly allocated to receive either an experimental intervention or some comparison management: usual treatment, a placebo, or simple observation. On the average, the compared groups have a similar prognosis just after randomization (and before the interventions). However, differences not attributable to treatment can arise later, including not taking the assigned treatment, dropping out of the study, receiving the other treatment, being managed differently in other ways, or getting treatments that are not part of the study. Blinding all participants in the trial can help minimize bias in how patients are randomized, managed, and assessed for outcomes but is not always possible or successful.

The results of randomized trials can be summarized according to the treatment assigned; an intention-to-treat analysis, which is a test of the clinical decision and maintains a randomized trial design; or according to the treatment actually received, which bears on the biology of disease, but not directly on the clinical decision, and has the disadvantage that patients may not remain with the treatment they were originally assigned. To obtain information more closely tailored to individual patients than the main results of randomized trials afford, clinicians can use results in subgroups of patients, which carry the additional risk of being misleading, or do trials on their own patients, one at a time.

For many clinical questions it is not possible, or not practical, to rely on a randomized controlled trial. Compromises with the ideal include making comparisons to experience with past patients, to past experience with the same patients, or to a concurrent group of patients who are not randomly allocated. When these compromises are done, the internal validity of the study is weakened.

REFERENCES

1. EC/IC Bypass Study Group. Failure of extracranial-intracranial arterial bypass to reduce the risk of ischemic stroke. N Engl J Med 1985;313:1191–1200.
2. Mayberg MR, Wilson E, Yatsu F, Weiss DG, Messina L, Hershey LA, Colling C, Eskridge J, Deykin D, Winn HR. Carotid endarterectomy and prevention of cerebral ischemia in symptomatic carotid stenosis. JAMA 1991;266:3289–3294.
3. Opie on the heart [Editorial]. Lancet 1980;1:692.
4. Rubenstein LZ, Robbins AS, Josephson KR, Schulman BL, Osterweil D. The value of assessing falls in an elderly population. A randomized controlled trial. Ann Intern Med 1990;113:308–316.
5. Fischer RW. Comparison of antipruritic drugs administered orally. JAMA 1968;203:418–419.

6. Ziegler EJ, et al. Treatment of gram negative bacteremia and septic shock with HA-1A human monoclonal antibody against endotoxin. New Engl J Med 1991;324:429–436.

7. Coronary Drug Project Research Group. Influence of adherence to treatment and response of cholesterol on mortality in the coronary drug project. N Engl J Med 1980;303:1038–1041.

8. Lipid Research Clinics Program. The Lipid Research Clinics coronary primary prevention trial results. 1. Reduction in incidence of coronary heart disease. JAMA 1984;251:351–364.

9. Byington RP, et al. Assessment of double-blindness at the conclusion of the beta-blocker heart attack trial. JAMA 1985;253:1733–1736.

10. Laupacis A, Sackett DL, Roberts RS. An assessment of clinically useful measures of the consequences of treatment. New Engl J Med 1988;318:1728–1733.

11. Naylor CD, Chen E, Strauss B. Measured enthusiasm: does the method of reporting trial results alter perceptions of therapeutic effectiveness? Ann Intern Med 1992;117:916–921.

12. Malenka DJ, Baron JA, Johansen S, Wahrenberger JW, Ross JM. The framing effect of relative and absolute risk. J Gen Intern Med 1993;8:543–548.

13. McNeil BJ, Pauker SG, Sox HC Jr, Tversky A. On the elicitation of preferences for alternative therapies.. New Engl J Med 1982;306:1259.

14. Sackett DL, Gent M. Controversy in counting and attributing events in clinical trials. N Engl J Med 1979;301:1410–1412.

15. Steering Committee of the Physicians' Health Study Research Group. Final report of the aspirin component of the ongoing Physicians' Health Study. New Engl J Med 1989;321:129–135.

16. Guyatt G, Sackett D, Taylor DW, Chong J, Roberts R, Pugsley S. Determining optimal therapy—randomized trials in individual patients. N Engl J Med 1986;314:889–892.

17. Feinstein AR, Sosin DM, Wells CK. The Will Rogers phenomenon. Stage migration and new diagnostic techniques as a source of misleading statistics for survival in cancer. New Engl J Med 1985;312:1604–2608.

18. Sacks H, Chalmers TC, Smith H Jr. Randomized versus historical controls for clinical trials. Am J Med 1982;72:233–240.

19. Topol EJ, Califf RM. Scorecard cardiovascular medicine. Its impact and future direction. Ann Intern Med 1994;120:65–70.

20. Ropes M. Systemic lupus erythematosus. Cambridge, MA: Havard University Press, 1976.

21. Spilker B. Guide to clinical interpretation of data. New York: Raven Press, 1986.

SUGGESTED READINGS

Chalmers TC, Smith H Jr, Blackburn B, Silverman B, Schroeder B, Reitman D, Ambroz A. A method for assessing the quality of a randomized control trial. Control Clin Trials 1981; 2:31–49.

Department of Clinical Epidemiology and Biostatistics, McMaster University, Hamilton, Ont. How to read clinical journals. V: To distinguish useful from useless or even harmful therapy. Can Med Assoc J 1981;124:1156–1162.

DerSimonian R, Charette LJ, McPeek B, Mosteller F. Reporting on methods in clinical trials. N Engl J Med 1982;306:1332–1337.

Feinstein AR. An additional basic science for clinical medicine. II: The limitations of randomized trials. Ann Intern Med 1983;99:544–550.

Friedman LM, Furberg CD, De Mets DL. Fundamentals of clinical trials. 2nd ed. Littleton, MA: John Wright PSG, 1985.

Guyatt GH, Sackett DL, Cook DJ. How to read clinical journals. II: How to use and article about therapy or prevention. A: Are the results of the study valid? JAMA 1993;270:2598–2601.

Guyatt GH, Sackett DL, Cook DJ. How to read clinical journals. II: How to use and article about therapy or prevention. B: What were the results and will they help me in caring for my patients? JAMA 1994;271:59–63.

Guyatt G, Sackett D, Taylor DW, Chong J, Roberts R, Pugsley S. Determining optimal therapy—randomized trials in individual patients. N Engl J Med 1986;314:889—892.

Hellman S, Hellman DS. Of mice and men. Problems of the randomized clinical trial. New Engl J Med 1991;324:1585–1589.

Laupakis A, Wells G, Richardson S, Tugwell P. Users' guide to the medical literature. V: How to use an article about prognosis. 1994;272:234–237.

Lavori PW, Louis TA, Bailar JC III, Polansky M. Design for experiments—parallel comparisons of treatment. N Engl J Med 1983;309:1291–1298.

Meinert CL. Clinical trials: design, conduct and analysis. New York: Oxford University Press, 1986.

Mostelller F, Gilbert JP, McPeek B. Reporting standards and research strategies for controlled trials. Control Clin Trials 1980;1:37–58.

Oxman AD, Guyatt GH. A consumer's guide to subgroup analysis. Ann Intern Med 1992;116:78–84.

Peto R, Pike MC, Armitage P, Breslow NE, Cox DR, Howard SV, Mantel N, McPherson K, Peto J, Smith PG. Design and analysis of randomized clinical trials requiring prolonged observation of each patient, part 1. Br J Cancer, 1976;34:585–612.

Peto R, Pike MC, Armitage P, Breslow NE, Cox DR, Howard SV, Mantel N, McPherson K, Peto J, Smith PG. Design and analysis of randomized clinical trials requiring prolonged observation of each patient, part 2. Br J Cancer, 1977;35:1–39.

Pocock SJ. Clinical trials: a practical approach. New York; John Wiley & Sons, 1983.

Yusuf S, Collins R, Peto R. Why do we need some large, simple randomized trials? Stat Med 1984;3:409–420.

8

PREVENTION

Live sensibly—among a thousand people, only one dies a natural death, the rest succumb to irrational modes of living.
Maimonides 1135–1204 A.D.

Most doctors are attracted to medicine because they look forward to curing disease. But all things considered, most patients would prefer never to contract a disease in the first place—or, if they cannot avoid an illness, they prefer that it be caught early and stamped out before it causes them any harm. To accomplish this, procedures are performed on patients without specific complaints, to identify and modify risk factors to avoid the onset of disease or to find disease early in its course so that by intervening patients can remain well. Such activity is referred to as *health maintenance* or *the periodic health examination*.

Health maintenance constitutes a large portion of clinical practice (1). Often, health maintenance activities can be incorporated into the ongoing care of patients, as when a doctor checks the blood pressure in a patient complaining of a sore throat; sometimes, a special visit just for health maintenance is scheduled.

Physicians should understand the conceptual basis and content of the periodic health examination. They should be prepared to answer questions from patients such as "Why do I have to get a Pap smear again this year, Doctor?" or "My neighbor gets a chest x-ray every year; why aren't you ordering one for me?"

This chapter concentrates on prevention activities clinicians undertake with individual patients. However, prevention at the community level is also effective. Immunization requirements for students, no-smoking regulations in public buildings, and legislation restricting the sale of firearms are examples of communitywide prevention. For some problems, such as injury prevention from firearms, community prevention works best. For others, such as colorectal cancer, screening in clinical settings works best. For still others, clinical efforts can complement communitywide activities, as in smoking prevention efforts by which clinicians help individual patients stop smoking and public education, regulations, and taxes prevent teenagers from starting to smoke.

Much of the scientific approach to prevention in clinical medicine, particularly the principles underlying the use of a diagnostic tests, disease prognosis, and effectiveness of interventions, has already been covered in this book. This chapter expands on those principles and strategies as they specifically relate to prevention.

Levels of Prevention

Webster's (2) dictionary defines prevention as "the act of keeping from happening." With this definition in mind, almost all activities in medicine could be defined as prevention. After all, clinicians' efforts are aimed at preventing the untimely occurrences of death, disease, disability, discomfort, dissatisfaction, and destitution (Chapter 1). However, in clinical medicine, the definition of prevention is usually restricted, as outlined below. Although more prevention is practiced than ever before, clinicians still spend most of their time in diagnosing and treating rather than in preventing disease.

Depending on when in the course of disease interventions are made, three types of prevention are possible (Fig. 8.1).

PRIMARY PREVENTION

Primary prevention keeps disease from occurring at all, by removing its causes. Folic acid administration to prevent neural tube defects, immunizations for many communicable diseases, and counseling patients to adopt healthy lifestyles (e.g., helping patients to stop smoking, to eat foods low in saturated fats and cholesterol and high in fiber, to exercise appropriately, and to engage in safe sexual practices) are examples of primary prevention.

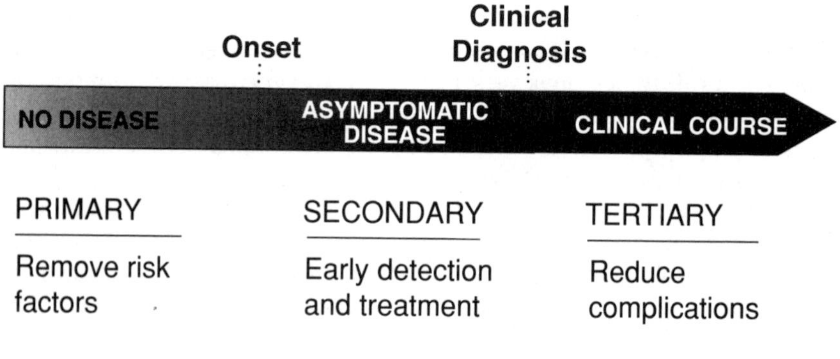

Figure 8.1. Levels of prevention.

Primary prevention is often accomplished outside the health care system at the community level, as noted above. Chlorination and fluoridation of the water supply and laws mandating seat belt use in automobiles and helmets for motorcycle use are examples. Certain primary prevention activities occur in specific occupational settings (use of ear plugs or dust masks), in schools (immunizations), or in specialized health care settings (use of tests to detect the hepatitis B or HIV in blood donations in blood banks).

SECONDARY PREVENTION

Secondary prevention detects disease early when it is asymptomatic and when early treatment can stop it from progressing; Pap smears, mammograms, and fecal occult blood tests are examples. Most secondary prevention is done in clinical settings, and all physicians, especially those caring for adults, undertake secondary prevention. There are a few community-wide programs (shopping mall fairs for glaucoma screening are an example).

SCREENING

Screening is the identification of an unrecognized disease or risk factor by history taking (e.g., asking if the patient smokes), physical examination (e.g., a prostate examination), laboratory test (e.g., a serum phenylalanine determination), or other procedure (e.g., a sigmoidoscopy) that can be applied rapidly. Screening tests sort out apparently well persons who have a disease or a risk factor for a disease from those who do not. It is part of many primary and all secondary prevention activities. A screening test is not intended to be diagnostic. If the clinician is not committed to further investigation of abnormal results and treatment, if necessary, the screening test should not be performed at all.

TERTIARY PREVENTION

Tertiary prevention refers to those clinical activities that prevent further deterioration or reduce complications after a disease has declared itself. An example is the use of beta-blocking drugs to decrease the risk of death in patients who have recovered from myocardial infarction. The boundaries of tertiary prevention blend into curative medicine, but well-performed tertiary prevention goes beyond treating the problems patients present with. For example, in diabetic patients, tertiary prevention requires more than good control of blood glucose; patients need regular ophthalmologic examinations for early diabetic retinopathy, education for routine foot care, searches for and treatment of other cardiovascular risk factors, and monitoring for urinary protein so that angiotensin-converting enzyme inhibitors can be used to prevent renal failure.

Tertiary prevention is particularly important in the management of patients with fatal disease. The goal here is not to prevent death but to maximize the amount of high-quality time a patient has left. For example, presently there is no specific therapy for patients with amyotrophic lateral sclerosis, a neurologic condition ending in paralysis of respiratory and swallowing muscles. But careful medical management can lead to early intervention with a gastrostomy for administering food and liquids to prevent dehydration and weakness from starvation, a tracheostomy for better suctioning to prevent pneumonia for as long as possible, and if the patient wishes, a portable respirator to rest respiratory muscles. Without such a proactive approach, the patient may present with acute respiratory failure due to the combined effects of the underlying disease, dehydration, and pneumonia. Patient, family, and physician are then faced with endotracheal intubation and admission to the intensive care unit, with the hope of reversing enough of the processes to reestablish decent quality of life for a little longer. Tertiary prevention can help avoid this scenario.

There are few, if any, tertiary prevention programs outside the health care system, but many health care professionals in addition to physicians are active in these programs.

Approach to the Periodic Health Examination

When considering what to do routinely for patients without specific symptoms for a given disease, the clinician must first decide which medical problems or diseases he or she should try to prevent. This statement is so straightforward that it would seem unnecessary. But the fact is that many preventive procedures, especially screening tests, are performed without a clear understanding of what is being sought. For instance, a urinalysis is frequently ordered by physicians performing routine checkups on their patients. However, a urinalysis might be used to search for any number of medical problems, including diabetes, asymptomatic urinary tract infections, and renal calculi. It is necessary to decide which, if any, of these conditions is worth screening for before undertaking the test.

Three criteria are important when deciding what condition to include in a periodic health examination (Table 8.1): (a) the burden of suffering caused by the condition, (b) the quality of screening test if one is to be performed, and (c) the effectiveness of the intervention for primary prevention (e.g., counseling patients to practice safe sex) or the effectiveness of treatment for secondary prevention after the condition is found on screening (e.g., prostate cancer treatment).

Burden of Suffering

Is screening justified by the severity of the medical condition in terms of mortality, morbidity, and suffering caused by the condition? Only conditions posing threats to life or health (the six Ds) should be sought. The severity of the medical condition is determined primarily by the risk it

Table 8.1
Criteria for Deciding Whether a Medical Condition Should Be Included in Periodic Health Examinations

1. How great is the burden of suffering caused by the condition in terms of:
   Death   Discomfort
   Disease   Dissatisfaction
   Disability   Destitution
2. How good is the screening test, if one is to be performed, in terms of:
   Sensitivity   Cost   Labeling effects
   Specificity   Safety
   Simplicity   Acceptability
3. a. For primary prevention, how effective is the intervention?
      or
   b. For secondary prevention, if the condition is found, how effective is the ensuing treatment in terms of:
      Efficacy
      Patient compliance
      Early treatment being more effective than later treatment

poses or its prognosis (discussed in Chapters 5 and 6). For example, except during pregnancy and before urologic surgery, the health consequences of asymptomatic bacteriuria are not clear. We do not know if it causes renal failure and/or hypertension. Even so, bacteriuria is frequently sought in periodic health examinations.

Burden of suffering takes into account the frequency of a condition. Often a particular condition causes great suffering for individuals unfortunate enough to get it, but occurs too rarely—perhaps in the individual's particular age group—for screening to be considered. Breast cancer and colorectal cancer are two such examples. Although both can occur in much younger people, they primarily occur in persons older than 50 years. For women in their early 20s, breast cancer incidence is 1 in 100,000 (one-fifth the rate for men in their early 70s) (3). Although breast cancer should be sought in periodic health examinations in women over 50, it is too uncommon in 20-year-old women (or 70-year-old men) for screening. Screening for very rare diseases means not only that at most very few people will benefit but, because of false-positive tests, that many people may suffer harm from labeling and further workup (see below).

A particularly difficult dilemma faced by clinicians and patients is the situation in which a person is known to be at high risk for a condition, but there is no evidence that early treatment is effective. What should the physician and patient do? For example, there is evidence that people with Barrett's esophagus (a condition in which the squamous mucosa in the distal esophagus is replaced by columnar epithelium) run a 30- to 40-fold greater risk of developing esophageal cancer than persons without Barrett's esophagus (4). However, the effectiveness of screening such people with periodic endoscopic examinations followed by early treatment if cancer occurs is unknown.

There is no easy answer to this dilemma. But if physicians remember that screening will not work unless early therapy is effective, they can weigh carefully the evidence about therapy with the patient. If the evidence is against effectiveness, they may hurt rather than help the patient by screening.

Which Tests?

The following criteria for a good screening test apply to all types of screening tests, whether they are history, physical examination, laboratory tests or procedures.

SENSITIVITY AND SPECIFICITY

The very nature of searching for a disease in people without symptoms for the disease means prevalence is usually very low, even among high-risk groups selected because of age, sex, and other characteristics. A good screening test must, therefore, have a high sensitivity, so it does not miss the few cases of disease that are present, and a high specificity, to reduce the number of people with false-positive results who require further workup.

Sensitivity and specificity are determined for screening tests much as they are for diagnostic tests, except that the gold standard for the presence of disease usually is not another test but rather a period of follow-up. For example, in a study of fecal occult blood tests for colorectal cancer, the sensitivity of the test was determined by the ratio of the number of colorectal cancers found during screening to that number plus the number of *interval cancers*, colorectal cancers subsequently discovered over the following year in the people with negative test results (the assumption being that interval cancers were present at screening but were missed, i.e., the test results were false negative) (5). Determination of sensitivity and specificity for screening tests in this way is sometimes referred to as the *detection method*.

The detection method for calculating sensitivity works well for many screening tests, but there are two difficulties with the method for some cancer screening tests. First, it requires that the appropriate amount of follow-up time is known; often it is not known and must be guessed. The method also requires that the abnormalities detected by the screening test would go on to cause trouble if left alone. This second issue is a problem in screening for prostate cancer. Because histologic prostate cancer is so common in men (it is estimated that 25% of 50-year-old men have histologic foci of prostate cancer, and by the age of 90, virtually all men do), screening tests can find such cancers in many men, but for most, the cancer will never become malignant. Thus, when the sensitivity of prostate cancer tests such as prostate-specific antigen (PSA) is determined by the detection method, the test may look quite good, since the numerator includes all cancers found, not just those with malignant potential.

To get around these problems, the *incidence method,* a new method, calculates sensitivity by using the incidence in persons not undergoing screening and the interval cancer rate in persons who are screened. The rationale for this approach is that the sensitivity of a test should affect interval cancer rates but not disease incidence. For prostate cancer, the incidence method defines sensitivity of the test as 1 minus the ratio of the interval prostate cancer rate in a group of men undergoing periodic screening to the incidence of prostate cancer in a group of men not undergoing screening (control group). The incidence method of calculating sensitivity gets around the problem of counting "benign" prostate cancers, but it may underestimate sensitivity because it excludes cancers with long lead times. True sensitivity of a test is, therefore, probably between the estimates of the two methods.

Because of the low prevalence of most diseases, the positive predictive value of most screening tests is low, even for tests with high specificity. Clinicians who practice preventive health care by performing screening tests on their patients must accept the fact that they will have to work up many patients who will not have disease. However, they can minimize the problem by concentrating their screening efforts on people with a higher prevalence for disease.

> **Example**   The incidence of breast cancer increases with age, from approximately 1 in 100,000/year at age 20 to 1 in 200/year over age 70. Therefore, a lump found during screening in a young woman's breast is more likely to be nonmalignant than a lump in an older woman. In a large demonstration project on breast cancer screening, biopsy results of breast masses varied markedly according to the age of women (6); in women under age 40, more than 16 benign lesions were found for every malignancy, but in women over age 70 fewer than 3 benign lesions were found for every malignancy (Fig. 8.2). Sensitivity and specificity of the clinical breast examination and mammography are better in older women as well, because of changes in breast tissue as women grow older.

The yield of screening decreases as screening is repeated over time in a group of people. Figure 8.3 demonstrates why this is true. The first time that screening is carried out—the *prevalence screen*—cases of the medical condition will have been present for varying lengths of time. During the second round of screening, most cases found will have had their onset between the first and second screening. (A few will have been missed by the first screen.) Therefore, second and subsequent screenings are called *incidence screens.* Figure 8.3 illustrates how, when a group of people are

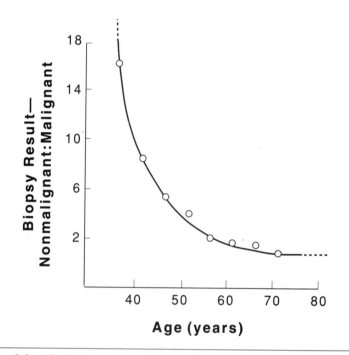

Figure 8.2. Yield of a screening test according to patients' age. Ratio of nonmalignant:malignant biopsy results among women screened for breast cancer. (Data from Baker LH. Breast Cancer Detection Demonstration Project: five-year summary report. CA 1982;32:195–231.)

periodically rescreened, the number of cases of disease present in the group drops after the prevalence screen. This means that the positive predictive value for test results will decrease after the first round of screening.

SIMPLICITY AND LOW COST

An ideal screening test should take only a few minutes to perform, require minimum preparation by the patient, depend on no special appointments, and be inexpensive.

Simple, quick examinations such as blood pressure determinations are ideal screening tests. Conversely, complicated diagnostic tests such as colonoscopy, which are expensive and require an appointment and bowel preparation, are reasonable in patients with symptoms and clinical indications but may be unacceptable as screening tests, especially if they must be repeated frequently. Other tests, such as visual field testing for the detection of glaucoma and audiograms for the detection of hearing loss, fall between these two extremes. Even if done carefully, such tests, al-

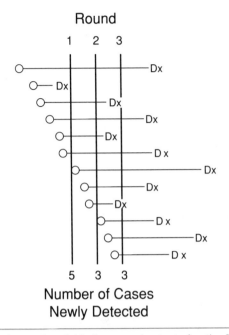

Figure 8.3.   The decreasing yield of a screening test after the first round of screening. The first round (prevalence screening) detects prevalent cases. The second and third rounds (incidence screenings) detect incident cases. It is assumed that the test detects all cases and that all people in the population are screened. If not, cases not detected in the first round are available for detection in subsequent rounds— and the yield can be higher. *Dx*, diagnosis.

though not as difficult as colonoscopy, are probably too complex to be used as screening tests.

The financial "cost" of the test depends not only on the cost of (or charge for) the procedure itself but also on the cost of subsequent evaluations performed on patients with positive test results. Thus sensitivity, specificity, and predictive value affect cost. Cost is also affected by whether the test requires a special visit to the physician. Screening tests performed while the patient is seeing his or her physician for other reasons (as is frequently the case with blood pressure measurements) are much cheaper for patients than tests requiring special visits, extra time off from work, and additional transportation.

SAFETY

It is reasonable and ethical to accept a certain risk for diagnostic tests applied to sick patients seeking help for specific complaints. The patient comes asking for help, sometimes with a problem about which little is known.

The physician cannot postpone action and does his or her best. It is quite another matter to subject presumably well people to risks when there is no known problem. In such circumstances, the procedure should be especially safe. This is partly because the chances of finding disease in healthy people are so low. Thus, although colonoscopy is hardly thought of as a "dangerous" procedure when used on patients with gastrointestinal complaints, it may be too dangerous to use as a screening procedure because of the possibility of bowel perforation. In fact, if colonoscopy, with a perforation rate of 0.2%, were used to screen for colorectal cancer in women in their 50s, almost two perforations would occur for every cancer found. For women in their 70s, the ratio would reverse, because colorectal cancer is so much more common (7).

ACCEPTABLE TO BOTH PATIENTS AND CLINICIANS

The importance of acceptability is illustrated by experience with tests for early cervical cancer and early colon cancer. Women at greatest risk for cervical cancer are least likely to get routine Pap smears. The same problem holds true for colorectal cancer. Studies indicate there is a strong reluctance among asymptomatic North Americans to submit to periodic examinations of their lower gastrointestinal tracts—a finding that should be no surprise to any of us!

Table 8.2 shows acceptance of screening for colorectal cancer by various kinds of people. People who voluntarily attended a colorectal cancer screening clinic were very cooperative; they were willing to collect stool samples, smear the samples on guaiac-impregnated paper slides, and mail the slides to their doctors for clinical testing. Patients who did not volunteer were less willing to participate. Older persons, who are at greatest risk for colorectal cancer because of their age, were least willing to be screened.

Table 8.2
Patients' Acceptance of Screening Tests: Reported Response Rates for Returning Guaiac-impregnated Slides in Different Settings[a]

Setting	Participants Returning Slides (Percent)
Colorectal cancer screening program	85
Breast cancer screening program	70
HMO members aged 50–74 years	27
HMO members aged 50–74 years sent kit, reminder letter, and self-help booklet and who were called with instructions and reminders	48*

[a] Data from Myers RE, Ross EA, Wolf TA, Balshem A, Jepson C, Millner L. Behavioral interventions to increase adherence in colorectal screening. Med Care 1991;29:1039–1050; and Fletcher SW, Dauphinee WD. Should colorectal carcinoma be sought in periodic health examinations? An approach to the evidence. Clin Invest Med 1981;4:23–31.

Substantial extra effort can result in getting more people (but still fewer than half) to participate.

The acceptability of the test to clinicians is a criterion usually overlooked by all but the ones performing it. After one large, well-conducted study on the usefulness of screening, sigmoidoscopy was abandoned because the physicians performing the procedure—gastroenterologists, at that—found it too cumbersome and time-consuming to be justified by the yield (8). (Patient acceptance, 38%, was not good either.)

LABELING

The *labeling* effect describes the psychological effect of test results or diagnoses on patients. Studies of labeling suggest that test results can sometimes have important psychological effects on patients.

Labeling can either help or hurt patients. A positive labeling effect may occur when a patient is told that all the screening test results were normal. Most clinicians have heard such responses as, "Great, that means I can keep working for another year." If being given a clean bill of health promotes a positive attitude toward one's daily activities, a positive labeling effect has occurred.

On the other hand, being told that something is abnormal may have an adverse psychological effect. A study of women who had false-positive mammograms (women with suspicious mammograms who on subsequent evaluation were found not to have cancer) found that several months later almost half reported mammography-related anxiety (47%) and worries about breast cancer (41%); 17% said the worries affected their daily function (9).

Labeling effects of screening tests may become a major concern with progress made in genetic screening. A gene has been identified for Huntington's chorea, and relatives of affected individuals can be tested to see if they carry the dominant, universally fatal gene. Such a test may help people who wonder if they should marry and have children. More complicated are the much more common situations in which genes are associated with a risk, not a certainty, of future disease. For example, several genes are known to be associated with colorectal and breast cancer. In these situations, many people with the genes will not get cancer, and many without the particular genes will get the cancer. Because the events are in the future, persons who have been told they have one of these genes will have to live with the possibility of a dire event for a long time.

Negative labeling effects are particularly worrisome ethically when they occur among patients with false-positive tests. In such situations, screening efforts might promote a sense of vulnerability instead of health and might do more harm than good.

RISK OF A FALSE-POSITIVE RESULT

The previous discussion applies to each of the individual screening tests that a clinician might consider performing during a periodic health examination. However, most clinicians do not perform only one or two tests on patients presenting for routine checkups. In one study, practicing internists believed that 57 different tests should be performed during periodic health examinations (10). Modern technology, and perhaps the threat of lawsuit, has fueled this propensity to "cover all the bases." Automated blood tests allow physicians to order up to several dozen tests with a few checks in the appropriate boxes.

When the measurements of screening tests are expressed on interval scales (as most are) and when *normal* is defined by the range covered by 95% of the results (as is usual), the more tests the clinician orders, the greater the risk of a false-positive result. In fact, as Table 8.3 shows, if the physician orders enough tests, "abnormalities" will be discovered in virtually all healthy patients.

Effectiveness of Treatment

"Treatments" in primary prevention are immunizations, such as tetanus toxoid to prevent tetanus; drugs, such as aspirin to prevent myocardial infarction; and behavioral counseling, such as helping patients stop smoking or adopt low-cholesterol diets. Whatever the intervention, it should be efficacious (produce a beneficial result in ideal situations) and effective (produce a beneficial result under usual conditions). Efficacy and effectiveness of pharmaceuticals are usually better documented than they are for behavioral counseling. Federal laws require rigorous evidence of efficacy before pharmaceuticals are approved for use. The same is not true for behavioral counseling methods, but clinicians should require scientific evidence before incorporating routine counseling into health maintenance. Health behaviors are among the most important determinants of health in modern society; effective counseling methods could promote health more

Table 8.3
Relation between Number of Tests Ordered and Percentage of Normal People with at Least One Abnormal Test Result[a]

Number of Tests	People with at Least One Abnormality (Percent)
1	5
5	23
20	64
100	99.4

[a] From Sackett DL. Clinical diagnosis and the clinical laboratory. Clin Invest Med 1978; 1:37–43.

than most anything else a clinician can do, but counseling that does not work wastes time, costs money, and may harm patients.

Example Two different smoking cessation counseling strategies— weekly hour-long group counseling sessions for 8 weeks and weekly 10- to 20-min individual counseling sessions for 8 weeks—were combined with nicotine patch therapy and evaluated for their effectiveness in promoting smoking cessation (11,12). Compared with patients randomized to control groups, the patients receiving the interventions did somewhat better, with a third of patients in the group counseling sessions having stopped smoking at 6 months follow-up. However, fewer than 20% of patients receiving individual counseling had stopped smoking. Furthermore, the authors found that most failures at 6 months could be predicted by patients smoking at some time during the first 2 weeks after trying to stop. These findings suggest that counseling should be "front loaded." By carefully evaluating behavioral counseling, studies such as this are determining what approaches work.

Treatments for secondary prevention are generally the same as treatments for curative medicine. Like interventions for primary prevention, they should be both efficacious and effective. If early treatment is not effective, it is not worth screening for a medical problem regardless of how easily it can be found, because early detection alone merely extends the length of time the disease is known to exist, without helping the patient.

Another criterion important for treatments in secondary prevention is that patient outcome must be better if the disease is found by screening, when it is asymptomatic, than when it is discovered later, after the condition becomes symptomatic and the person seeks medical care. If outcome in the two situations is the same, screening is not necessary.

Example In a study of the use of chest x-rays and sputum cytology to screen for lung cancer, male cigarette smokers who were screened every 4 months and treated promptly if cancer was found did no better than those not offered screening (13); at the end of the study, death rates from lung cancer were the same in the two groups—3.2 per 1000 person-years in the screened men versus 3.0 per 1000 persons-years in men not offered screening. Early detection and treatment did not help patients with lung cancer more than treatment of people at the time they presented with symptoms.

BIASES

As discussed in Chapter 7, the best way to establish the efficacy of treatment is with a randomized controlled trial. This is true for all interventions but especially for early treatment after screening. To establish that a preventive intervention is effective typically takes years and requires large numbers of people to be studied. For example, early treatment after colorectal cancer screening can decrease colorectal cancer deaths by approximately one-third. But to show this effect, a study with 13 years of follow-up was required (5). A "clinical impression" of the effect of screening simply does not suffice in this situation.

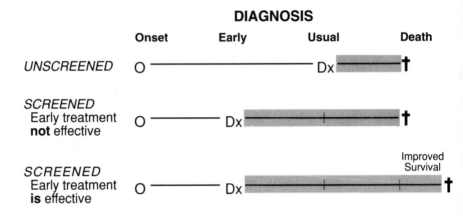

Figure 8.4. How lead time affects survival time after screening; shaded areas indicate length of survival after diagnosis (Dx).

Careful studies are also necessary because of biases that are specific to studies of the effectiveness of screening programs. Three such biases are described below.

Lead Time Bias

Lead time is the period of time between the detection of a medical condition by screening and when it ordinarily would be diagnosed because a patient experiences symptoms and seeks medical care (Fig. 8.4). The amount of lead time for a given disease depends on both the biologic rate of progression of the disease and on the ability of the screening test to detect early disease. When lead time is very short, as is presently the case with lung cancer, treatment of medical conditions picked up on screening is likely to be no more effective than treatment after symptoms appear. On the other hand, when lead time is long, as is true for cervical cancer (on average, it takes approximately 30 years to progress from carcinoma in situ to clinically invasive disease), treatment of the medical condition found on screening can be very effective.

How can lead time cause biased results in a study of the efficacy of early treatment? As Figure 8.4 shows, because of screening, a disease is found earlier than it would have been after the patient developed symptoms. As a result, people who are diagnosed by screening for a deadly disease will, on average, survive longer from the time of diagnosis than people who are diagnosed after they get symptoms, even if early treatment is no more effective than treatment at clinical presentation. In such a situation screening would appear to help people live longer, when in a reality they would be given not more "survival time" but more "disease time."

Screening

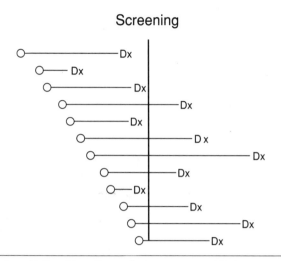

Figure 8.5.   Length time bias. Cases that progress rapidly from onset (O) to symptoms and diagnosis (Dx) are less likely to be detected during a screening examination.

An appropriate method of analysis to avoid lead time bias is to study both a screened group of people and a control group of people and compare age-specific mortality rates rather than survival rates from the time of diagnoses. We can be confident that early diagnoses and treatment of colorectal cancer are effective, because studies have shown that mortality rates of screened persons are lower than those of a comparable group of unscreened people (5).

Length Time Bias

Length time bias (see Figs. 8.5 and 8.6), another bias that can affect studies of screening, occurs because the proportion of slow-growing lesions diagnosed during screening programs is greater than the proportion of those diagnosed during usual medical care. The effect of including a greater number of slow-growing cancers makes it seem that screening and early treatment are more effective than usual care.

Length time bias occurs in the following way. Screening works best when a medical condition develops slowly. Most types of cancers, however, demonstrate a wide range of growth rates. Some cancers grow slowly, some very fast. Screening tests are likely to find mostly slow-growing tumors because they are present for a longer period of time before they cause symptoms; fast-growing tumors are more likely to cause symptoms that lead to diagnosis in the interval between screening examinations. Screening, therefore, tends to find tumors with inherently better prognoses. As a result, the mortality rates of cancers found on screening may be better than those not found on screening, but it is not because of the screening itself.

Compliance Bias

Compliance bias, the third major type of bias that can occur in effectiveness studies of presymptomatic treatment is the result of the extent to which patients follow medical advice. Compliant patients tend to have better prognoses regardless of screening. If a study compares disease outcomes among volunteers for a screening program with outcomes in a group of people who did not volunteer, better results for the volunteers might not be due to treatment but be the result of other factors related to compliance.

> ***Example*** In a study of the effect of a health maintenance program, one group of patients was invited for an annual periodic health examination and a comparable group was not invited (14). Over the years, however, some of the control group asked for periodic health examinations. As seen in Figure 8.7, those patients in the control group who actively sought out the examinations had better mortality rates than the patients who were invited for screening. The latter group contained not only compliant patients but also ones who had to be persuaded to participate.

Biases due to length time and patient compliance can be avoided by relying on randomized controlled trials that count all the outcomes in the groups, regardless of the method of diagnosis or degree of participation. Groups of patients that are randomly allocated will have comparable num-

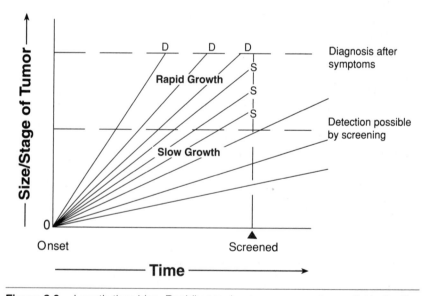

Figure 8.6. Length time bias. Rapidly growing tumors come to medical attention before screening is performed, whereas more slowly growing tumors allow time for detection. *D,* diagnosis after symptoms; *S,* diagnosis after screening.

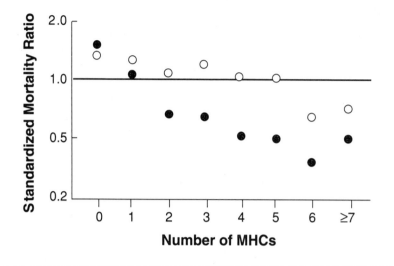

Figure 8.7. Effect of patient compliance on a screening program. The control group of patients (●) had a lower standardized mortality ratio (observed:expected deaths, standardized for age) than the study group offered (○) screening; but the control group included only patients who requested screening, whereas the study group included all patients offered screening. *MHCs*, multiphasic health checkups. (Redrawn from Friedman GD, Collen MF, Fireman BH. Multiphasic health checkup evaluation: a 16-year follow-up. J Chron Dis 1986;39:453–463.)

bers of slow- and fast-growing tumors and, on average, comparable levels of compliance. These groups then can be followed over time with mortality rates, rather than survival rates to avoid lead time bias.

Because randomized controlled trials are difficult to conduct, take so long, and are expensive, investigators sometimes try to use other kinds of studies, such as cohort studies (Chapter 5) or case control studies (Chapter 10), to investigate preventive maneuvers and effectiveness of treatment after screening.

> *Example* To test whether periodic screening with sigmoidoscopy reduces mortality from colorectal cancer within the reach of the sigmoidoscope, Selby et al. (15) investigated the frequency of screening sigmoidoscopy over the previous 10 years among patients dying of colorectal cancer and among well patients, matched for age and sex. To deal with lead time and length time biases, they investigated screening only in people who were known to have died (case group) or not to have died (control group) from colorectal cancer. To deal with compliance bias, they adjusted their results for the number of general periodic health examinations each person had. They also adjusted the results for the presence of medical conditions that could have led to both increased screening and increased likelihood of colorectal cancer.

Patients dying of colorectal cancer in the rectum or distant sigmoid were less likely to have undergone a screening sigmoidoscopy in the previous 10 years (8.8%) than those in the control group (24.2%), and sigmoidoscopy followed by early therapy prevented almost 60% of deaths from distal colorectal cancer. Also, by showing that there was no protection for colorectal cancers above the level reached by sigmoidoscopy, the authors suggested that "it is difficult to conceive of how such anatomical specificity of effect could be explained by confounding."

Case series, in which a group of people participating in a screening program are followed over time, are a common but inappropriate method of evaluating the effectiveness of screening programs; they are subject to all the biases discussed (see Chapter 10 for more on case series).

How Much Harm for How Much Good?

Health promotion and disease prevention are becoming increasingly popular. The goal of keeping people as healthy as possible is laudable, but as this chapter points out, the concepts behind the goal are complex. Most important, health promotion activities can cause harm. In fact, it is probably fair to say that they usually do cause harm, even though totally unintended. At the least, they cost money, patients' time and often discomfort. At the worst, they can cause serious physical harm in the rare patient, either because of complications of the screening test itself or because of adverse consequences of subsequent tests or treatment, particularly in patients with false-positive test results. False-positive tests can cause psychological damage as well. Thus it is important that the clinician have solid evidence about how much good and how much harm health promotion activities accomplish. Good intentions are not enough.

Before undertaking a health promotion procedure on a patient, especially if the procedure is controversial among expert groups, the clinician should discuss both the pros (probability of known and hoped-for health benefits) and cons (probability of unintended effects) of the procedure with the patient.

> *Example* Although clinical breast examinations and mammography screening for breast cancer are universally recommended for older women, there is controversy about screening for women ages 40 to 49; randomized controlled trials show that screening does not work well in this age group, but a protective effect of about 15% may still be possible after many years. Expert groups are divided in their recommendations. When discussing this dilemma with a patient, it is useful to demonstrate both benefits and harms resulting from screening (Fig 8.8). Such an approach not only is more honest with the patient but helps clarify the situation for her so that her consent for whatever is chosen is truly informed. Cost effectiveness analysis formalizes this approach for policymakers (16).

Screened   **Not Screened**

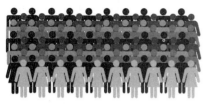   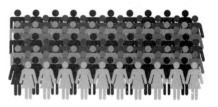

1000

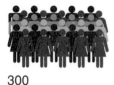

300   False-positive
mammograms

150   Procedures because
of mammograms

     New breast cancers

15   15

     Deaths from
breast cancer

5–8   7–8

Figure 8.8. Weighing benefit and harm from screening. What happens during a decade of annual mammography in 1000 women starting at age 40.

Current Recommendations

With progress in the science of prevention, current recommendations on health maintenance are quite different from those of the past. Several groups have recommended abandoning routine annual checkups in favor of a selective approach in which the tests to be done depend on a person's age, sex, and clinical characteristics (thereby increasing prevalence and positive predictive value). They have also tended to recommend fewer tests than previously (thereby decreasing the percentage of patients with false-positive results). Several groups have turned their attention to the selection process for deciding what medical conditions should be sought. There is increasing concern for clear delineation of the criteria that tests should meet before they are incorporated into periodic health examinations. Groups with explicit criteria for selecting medical conditions are more conservative in their recommendations than groups without such criteria.

Summary

Disease can be prevented by keeping it from occurring in the first place (primary prevention), with interventions such as immunization and behavioral counseling. Such interventions should be evaluated for effectiveness as rigorously as other kinds of clinical interventions.

Ill effects from disease can also be prevented by conducting screening tests at a time when presymptomatic treatment is more effective than treatment when symptoms occur (secondary prevention). A disease is sought if the disease causes a substantial burden of suffering, if a good screening test is available, and if presymptomatic treatment is more effective than treatment at the usual time. Screening tests should be sensitive enough to pick up most cases of the condition sought, specific enough that there are not too many false-positive results, inexpensive, safe, and well accepted by both patients and clinicians.

In secondary prevention, three potential biases threaten studies of the effectiveness of presymptomatic treatment: failure to account for the lead time gained by early detection, the tendency to detect a disproportionate number of slowly advancing cases when screening prevalent cases, and confounding the good prognosis associated with compliance with the effects of the preventive intervention itself.

Based on these criteria, a limited number of primary prevention interventions and screening tests for secondary prevention are recommended for health maintenance, according to the age, sex, and clinical status of the patient.

REFERENCES

1. Schappert SM. National ambulatory medical care survey: 1991 summary. Advance data from vital and health statistics. No. 230. Hyattsville, MD: National Center for Health Statistics, 1993.
2. Webster's ninth new collegiate dictionary. Springfield, MA: Merriam-Webster, 1991.
3. Ries LAG, Miller BA, Hankey BF, Kosary CL, Harras A, Edwards BK, eds. SEER cancer statistics review, 1973–1991: tables and graphs. NIH Publication No. 94–2789. Bethesda, MD: National Cancer Institute, 1994.
4. Cameron AJ, Ott BJ, Payne WS. The incidence of adenocarcinoma in columnar-lined (Barrett's) esophagus. N Engl J Med 1985;313:857–859.

5. Mandel JS, et al. Reducing mortality from colorectal cancer by screening for fecal occult blood. N Engl J Med 1993;328:1365–1371.
6. Baker LH. Breast Cancer Detection Demonstration Project: five-year summary report. CA 1982;32:195–231.
7. Eddy DM. Screening for colorectal cancer. Ann Intern Med 1990;113:373–384.
8. Dales LG, Friedman GD, Collen MF. Evaluating periodic multiphasic health check-ups: a controlled trial. J Chron Dis 1979;32:385–404.
9. Lerman C, Trock B, Rimer BK, Boyce A, Jepson C, Engstrom PF. Psychological and behavioral implications of abnormal mammograms. Ann Intern Med 1991;114:657–661.
10. Romm FJ, Fletcher SW, Hulka BS. The periodic health examination: comparison of recommendations and internists' performance. South Med J 1981;74:265–271.
11. Fiore MC, Kenford SL, Jorenby DE, Wetter DW, Smith SS, Baker TB. The nicotine patch: clinical effectiveness with different counseling treatments. Chest 1994;105:524–533.
12. Kenford, SL, Fiore MC, Jorenby DE, Smith SS, Wetter D, Baker TB. Predicting smoking cessation: who will quit with and without the nicotine patch. JAMA. 1994;271:589–594.
13. Fontana RS, Sanderson DR, Woolner LB, Taylor WF, Miller We, Muhm JR. Lung cancer screening: the Mayo program. J Occup Med 1986;28:746–750.
14. Friedman GD, Collen MF, Fireman BH. Multiphasic health checkup evaluation: a 16-year follow-up. J Chron Dis 1986;39:453–463.
15. Selby JV, Friedman GD, Quesenberry CP, Weiss NS. A case-control study of screening sigmoidoscopy and mortality from colorectal cancer. N Eng J Med 1992;326:653–657.
16. Eddy DM, Hasselblad V, McGivney W, Hendee W. The value of mammography screening in women under age 50 years. JAMA 1988;259:1512–1519.

SUGGESTED READINGS

Eddy DM (ed). Common screening tests. Philadelphia, American College of Physicians, 1991.
Goldbloom RB, Lawrence RS, eds, Preventing disease: beyond the rhetoric. New York: Springer-Verlag, 1990.
Guyatt GH, Sackett DL, Cook DJ. Users' guides to the medical literature. II: How to use an article about therapy or prevention. A: Are the results of the study valid? JAMA 1993;270:2598–2601.
Guyatt GH, Sackett DL, Cook DJ. Users' guides to the medical literature. II: How to use an article about therapy or prevention. B: What were the results and will they help me in caring for my patients? JAMA 1994;271:59–63.
Hayward RS, Steinberg EP, Ford DE, Roizen MF, Roach KW. Preventive care guidelines: 1991. Ann Intern Med 1991;114:758–783.
Miller AB, ed. Screening for cancer. Orlando, FL: Academic Press, 1985.
Miller AB, Chamberlain J, Day NE, Hakama M, Prorok PC, eds. Cancer screening. Cambridge, England: International Union Against Cancer, 1991.
Russell LB. Educated guesses: making policy about medical screening tests. Berkeley: University of California Press, 1994.
U.S. Preventive Services Task Force. Guide to preventive services: an assessment of the effectiveness of 169 interventions. Baltimore: Williams & Wilkins, 1989.

9

CHANCE

When clinicians attempt to learn from clinical experience, whether during formal research or in the course of patient care, their efforts are impeded by two processes: bias and chance. As we discussed (Chapter 1), bias is systematic error, the result of any process that causes observations to differ systematically from the true values. In clinical research, a great deal of the effort is aimed at avoiding bias where possible and controlling for and estimating its effects when bias is unavoidable.

Random error, on the other hand, is inherent in all observations. It can be minimized but never avoided altogether. Random variation can arise from the process of measurement itself or the biologic phenomenon being measured (Chapter 2). This source of error is called "random," because on average it is as likely to result in observed values being on one side of the true value as on the other.

Most of us tend to overestimate the importance of chance relative to bias when interpreting data. We might say, in essence, "If p is <0.001, a little bit of bias can't do much harm!" However, if data are assembled with unrecognized bias, no amount of statistical elegance can save the day. As one scholar put it, perhaps taking an extreme position, "A well designed, carefully executed study usually gives results that are obvious without a formal analysis and if there are substantial flaws in design or execution a formal analysis will not help" (1).

In this chapter, chance is discussed in the context of a controlled clinical trial, because that is a simple way of presenting the concepts. However, application of the concepts is not limited to comparisons of treatments in clinical trials. Statistics are used whenever one makes inferences about populations based on information obtained from samples.

Random Error

The observed differences between treated and control patients in a clinical trial cannot be expected to represent the true differences exactly because of random variation in both of the groups being compared. Statistical tests help estimate how well the observed difference approximates the true one. Why not measure the phenomenon directly and do away with this uncertainty? Because research must ordinarily be conducted on a sample of patients and not all patients with the condition under study. As a result, there is always a possibility that the particular sample of patients in a study, even though selected in an unbiased way, might not be similar to the population of patients as a whole.

Two general approaches are used to assess the role of chance in clinical observations. The first, called *hypothesis testing*, asks whether an effect (difference) is present or not by using statistical tests to examine the hypothesis that there is no difference (the "null hypothesis"). This is the traditional way of assessing the role of chance, popular since statistical testing was introduced at the beginning of this century and associated with the familiar "*p* values." The other approach, called *estimation*, uses statistical methods to estimate the range of values that is likely to include the true value. This approach has gained popularity recently and is now favored by most journals for reasons that we describe below.

We begin with a description of the traditional approach.

Hypothesis Testing

In the usual situation, where the principal conclusions of a trial are expressed in dichotomous terms (e.g., the treatment is considered to be either successful or not) and the results of the statistical test is also dichotomous (the result is either "statistically significant"—i.e., unlikely to be purely by chance—or not), there are four ways in which the conclusions of the test might relate to reality (Fig. 9.1).

Two of the four possibilities lead to correct conclusions: (a) when the treatments really do have different effects and that is the conclusion of the study and (b) when the treatments really have similar effects and the study makes that conclusion.

There are also two ways of being wrong. The treatments under study may actually have similar effects, but it is concluded that the study treatment is better. Error of this kind, resulting in the "false-positive" conclusion that the treatment is effective, is referred to as an α or *Type I* error. Alpha is the probability of saying that there is a difference in treatment effects when there is not. On the other hand, treatment might be effective, but the study concludes that it is not. This "false-negative" conclusion is called a β or *Type II* error. Beta is the probability of saying that there is no difference in treatment effects when there is one. "No difference" is a simplified way of saying that the true difference is unlikely to be larger than a certain size. It is not possible to establish that there is no difference at all between two treatments.

Figure 9.1 is similar to the two-by-two table comparing the results of a

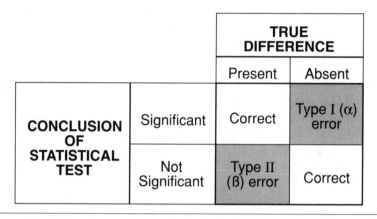

Figure 9.1. The relationship between the results of a statistical test and the true difference between two treatment groups. (*Absent* is a simplification. It really means that the true difference is not greater than a specified amount.)

diagnostic test to the true diagnosis (Chapter 3). Here the "test" is the conclusion of a clinical trial, based on a statistical test of results from a sample of patients. Reality is the true relative merits of the treatments being compared—if it could be established, for example, by making observations on all patients with the illness under study or a large number of samples of these patients. Alpha error is analogous to a false-positive and β error to a false-negative test result. In the absence of bias, random variation is responsible for the uncertainty of the statistical conclusion.

Because random variation plays a part in all observations, it is an oversimplification to ask whether or not chance is responsible for the results. Rather, it is a question of how likely random variation is to account for the findings under the particular conditions of the study. The probability of error due to random variation is estimated by means of *inferential statistics*, a quantitative science that, based on assumptions about the mathematical properties of the data, allows calculations of the probability that the results could have occurred by chance alone.

Statistics is a specialized field with its own jargon—null hypothesis, variance, regression, power, and modeling—that is unfamiliar to many clinicians. However, leaving aside the genuine complexity of statistical methods, inferential statistics should be regarded by the nonexpert as a useful means to an end. Statistical tests are the means by which the effects of random variation are estimated.

The next two sections discuss α and β error, respectively. We will attempt to place hypothesis testing, as it is used to estimate the probabilities of these errors, in context. However, we will make no attempt to deal with these subjects in a rigorous, quantitative fashion. For that, we suggest that readers consult any of a number of excellent textbooks of biostatistics (see "Suggested Readings," later in this chapter).

CONCLUDING THAT A TREATMENT WORKS

Most of the statistics encountered in the current medical literature concern the likelihood of an α error and are expressed by the familiar p value. The p value is a quantitative estimate of the probability that observed differences in treatment effects in the particular study at hand could have happened by chance alone, assuming that there is in fact no difference between the groups. Another way of expressing this is that p is an answer to the question, If there were no difference between treatments and the trial was repeated many times, what proportion of the trials would lead to the conclusion that a treatment is as or more effective than found in the study?

We will call the p value "p_α" to distinguish it from estimates of the other kind of error due to random variation, β error, which we will refer to as "p_β." When a simple p is found in the scientific literature it ordinarily refers to what we call p_α.

The kind of error estimated by p_α applies whenever it is concluded that one treatment is more effective than another. If it is concluded that the p_α exceeds some limit and so there is no difference between treatments, then the particular value of p_α is not as relevant; in that situation, p_β (probability of β error) applies.

DICHOTOMOUS AND EXACT p VALUES

It has become customary to attach special significance to p values falling below 0.05 because it is generally agreed that less than 1 chance in 20 is a small risk of being wrong. A rate of 1 in 20 is so small, in fact, that it is reasonable to conclude that such an occurrence is unlikely to have arisen by chance alone. It could have arisen by chance, and 1 in 20 times it will. But it is unlikely.

Differences associated with p_α less than 0.05 are called "statistically significant." It is important to remember, however, that setting a cutoff point at 0.05 is entirely arbitrary. Reasonable people might accept higher values or insist on lower ones, depending on the consequences of a false-positive conclusion in a given situation.

To accommodate various opinions about what is and is not unlikely enough, some researchers report the exact probabilities of p_αs (e.g., 0.03, 0.07, 0.11, etc.), rather than lumping them into two categories, <0.05 or >0.05. The interpretation of what is statistically significant is then left to the reader. However, p values greater than 1 in 5 are usually reported as simply $p > 0.20$, because nearly everyone can agree that a probability of an α error that is greater than one in five is unacceptably high. Similarly, below very low p values (such as $p < 0.001$) chance is a very unlikely explanation for the observed difference, and little further information is imparted by describing this chance more precisely.

STATISTICAL SIGNIFICANCE AND CLINICAL IMPORTANCE

A statistically significant difference, no matter how small the p, does not mean that the difference is clinically important. A $p < 0.0001$, if it emerges from a well-designed study, conveys a high degree of confidence that a difference really exists. But this p value tells us nothing about the magnitude of that difference or its clinical importance. In fact, entirely trivial differences may be highly statistically significant if a large enough number of patients was studied.

> *Example* In the early 1990s there was a heated debate about which thrombolytic agent, streptokinase or tissue plasminogen activator (tPA), is most effective during acute myocardial infarction. Large trials had shown a difference in reperfusion rates but not mortality. The two were compared (along with subcutaneous or intravenous heparin) in a large randomized controlled trial, called GUSTO, involving 41,021 patients in 15 countries (2). tPA was given by a more aggressive regimen than in earlier studies. The death rate at 30 days was lower among patients receiving tPA (6.3%) than among those receiving streptokinase (7.2 or 7.4%, depending on how heparin was given) and this difference was highly unlikely to be by chance ($p < 0.001$). However, the difference is not large; one would have to treat about 100 patients with tPA instead of with streptokinase to prevent one short-term death. Because tPA is much more expensive than streptokinase— it would cost nearly $250 thousand to prevent that death (3)—and because tPA is more likely to cause hemorrhagic strokes, some have questioned whether the marginal benefit of tPA is worthwhile, i.e., whether the difference in mortality between tPA and streptokinase treatment, all things considered, is "clinically significant."

On the other hand, very unimpressive p values can result from studies showing strong treatment effects if there are few patients in the study (see the following section).

STATISTICAL TESTS

Commonly used statistical tests, familiar to many readers, are used to estimate the probability of an α error. The tests are applied to the data to give a test statistic, which in turn can be used to come up with a probability of error (Fig. 9.2). The tests are of the *null hypothesis,* the proposition that there is no true difference in outcome between the two treatment groups. This device is for mathematical reasons, not because "no difference" is the working scientific hypothesis of the study. One ends up rejecting the null hypothesis (concluding there is a difference) or failing to reject it (concluding there is no difference).

Some commonly used statistical tests are listed in Table 9.1. The validity

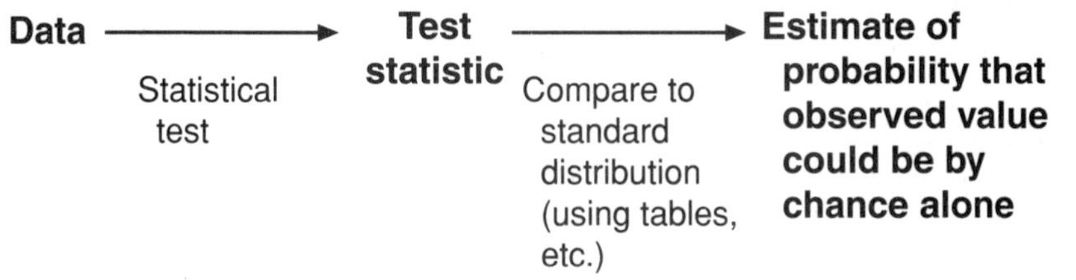

Data ——————————→ **Test** ——————————→ **Estimate of**

Statistical   **statistic** Compare to   **probability that**
test   standard   **observed value**
                              distribution   **could be by**
                              (using tables,   **chance alone**
                              etc.)

Figure 9.2. Statistical testing.

Table 9.1
Some Statistical Techniques Commonly Used in Clinical Research

To test the statistical significance of a difference	
Chi square (χ^2)	Between two or more proportions (when there is a large number of observations)
Fisher's exact	Between two proportions (when there is a small number of observations)
Mann-Whitney U	Between two medians
Student t	Between two means
F test	Between two or more means
To describe the extent of association	
Regression coefficient	Between an independent (predictor) variable and a dependent (outcome) variable
Pearson's r	Between two variables
To model the effects of multiple variables	
Logistic regression	On a dichotomous outcome
Cox proportional hazards	On a time-to-event outcome

of each test depends on certain assumptions about the data. If the data at hand do not satisfy these assumptions, the resulting p_α may be misleading. A discussion of how these statistical tests are derived and calculated and of the assumptions on which they rest can be found in any biostatistics textbook.

Example The chi square (χ^2) test, for nominal data (counts) is more easily understood than most and so can be used to illustrate how statistical testing works. Consider the following data from a randomized trial of two ways of initiating anticoagulation with heparin: a weight-based dosing nomogram and standard care (4). The outcome was a partial thromboplastin time (PTT) exceeding the therapeutic threshold within 24 hr of beginning anticoagulation. In the nomogram group 60 of 62 (97%) did so; in the standard care group, 37 of 48 (77%).

Observed Rates

	PTT Exceeding Threshold		
	Yes	No	Total
Nomogram	60	2	62
Standard care	37	11	48
Total	97	13	110

How likely would it be for a study of this size to observe a difference in rates as great as this or greater if there were in fact no differences in effectiveness? That depends on how far the observed results depart from what might have been expected if the treatments were of similar value and only random variation caused them to differ in the samples studied. If treatment had no effect on outcome, applying the success rate for the patients as a whole (88%) to the number of patients in each treatment group gives the expected number of successes in each group:

Expected Rates (Rounded to Nearest Integer)

	PTT Exceeding Threshold		
	Yes	No	Total
Nomogram	55	7	62
Standard care	42	6	48
Total	97	13	110

The χ^2 statistic, which quantitates the difference between the observed and expected numbers, is the sum for all four cells of:

$$\frac{(\text{Observed number} - \text{Expected number})^2}{\text{Expected number}}$$

The magnitude of the χ^2 statistic is determined by how different all of the observed numbers are from what would be expected if there were no treatment effect. Because they are squared, it does not matter whether the observed rates exceed or fall short of the expected. By dividing the squared difference in each cell by the expected number, the difference for that cell is adjusted for the number of patients in that cell.

The χ^2 statistic for these data is

$$\frac{(60 - 55)^2}{55} + \frac{(2 - 7)^2}{7} + \frac{(37 - 42)^2}{42} + \frac{(11 - 6)^2}{6} = 8.79$$

This χ^2 is then compared to a table relating χ^2 values to probabilities (available in books and computer programs) for that number of cells, to obtain the probability of a χ^2 that large or larger. It is intuitively obvious that the larger the χ^2, the less likely chance is to account for the observed differences. The result in this case is $p = 0.004$, which is the probability of a false-positive conclusion that the treatments had different effects.

CONCLUDING THAT A TREATMENT DOES NOT WORK

Some trials come to the conclusion that neither treatment is better than the other. There are some very influential examples, including studies showing that coronary artery bypass surgery does not prolong life in patients with chronic stable angina (except for those with left main coronary artery obstruction), that antioxidants do not prevent cancer, and that antibodies against endotoxin do not improve the prognosis of most patients with septic shock.

The question arises, could results like these have occurred by chance alone? Could the findings of such trials have misrepresented the truth because these particular studies had the bad luck to turn out in relatively unlikely ways? Specifically, what is the probability of a false-negative result (a β or Type II error)? The risk of a false-negative result is particularly large in studies with relatively few patients.

Beta error has received less attention than α error for several reasons. It is more difficult to calculate. Also, most of us simply prefer things that work. Negative results are unwelcome: authors are less likely to submit negative studies to journals and if negative studies are reported at all, the authors may prefer to emphasize subgroups of patients in which treatment differences are found, even if the differences are not statistically significant. Authors may also emphasize reasons other than chance for why true differences might have been missed. Whatever the reason for not considering the probability of β error, it is the main question that should be asked when the results of a study indicate no difference.

The probability that a trial will find a statistically significant difference when a difference really exists is called the *statistical power* of the trial.

$$\text{Statistical power} = 1 - p\beta$$

Power and $p\beta$ are complementary ways of expressing the same concept. Power is analogous to the sensitivity of a diagnostic test. In fact, one speaks of a study being powerful if it has a high probability of detecting as different treatments that really are different.

HOW MANY PATIENTS ARE ENOUGH?

Suppose you are reading about a clinical trial comparing a promising new therapy to the current form of treatment. You are aware that random variation can be the source of whatever differences are observed, and you wonder if the number of patients (*sample size*) in this study is large enough to make chance an unlikely explanation for what was found. How many patients would be necessary to make an adequate comparison of the effects of the two treatments? The answer depends on four characteristics of the study: the magnitude of the difference in outcome between treatment groups, p_α, p_β, and the nature of the study's data. These are taken into account when the researcher plans the study and when the reader decides whether the study has a reasonable chance of giving a useful answer.

Effect Size

Sample size depends on the magnitude of the difference to be detected. We are free to look for differences of any magnitude, and of course, we hope to be able to detect even very small differences. But more patients are needed to detect small differences, everything else being equal. So it is best to ask only that there is a sufficient number of patients to detect the smallest degree of improvement that would be clinically meaningful. On the other hand, if we are interested in detecting only very large differences between treated and control groups (i.e., strong treatment effects), then fewer patients need be studied.

Alpha Error

Sample size is also related to the risk of an α error (concluding that treatment is effective when it is not). The acceptable size for a risk of this kind is a value judgment; the risk could be as large as 1 or as small as 0. If one is prepared to accept the consequences of a large chance of falsely concluding that the therapy is valuable, one can reach conclusions with relatively few patients. On the other hand, if one wants to take only a small risk of being wrong in this way, a larger number of patients will be required. As we discussed earlier, it is customary to set p_α at 0.05 (1 in 20) or sometimes 0.01 (1 in 100).

Beta Error

The chosen risk of a β error is another determinant of sample size. An acceptable probability of this error is also a judgment that can be freely made and changed, to suit individual tastes. Probability of β is often set at 0.20, a 20% chance of missing true differences in a particular study. Conventional β errors are much larger than α errors, reflecting the higher value usually placed on being sure an effect is really present when we say it is.

Characteristics of the Data

The statistical power of a study is also determined by the nature of the data. When the outcome is expressed on a nominal scale and so is described by counts or proportions of events, its statistical power depends on the rate of events: the larger the number of events, the greater the statistical power for a given number of people at risk. As Peto et al. (5) put it,

> In clinical trials of time to death (or of the time to some other particular "event"—relapse, metastasis, first thrombosis, stroke, recurrence, or time to death from a particular cause), the ability of the trial to distinguish between the merits of two treatments depends on how many patients die (or suffer a relevant event), rather than on the number of patients entered. A study of 100 patients, 50 of whom die, is about as sensitive as a study with 1000 patients, 50 of whom die.

If the outcome is a continuous variable, such as blood pressure or serum cholesterol, power is affected by the degree to which patients vary among themselves: The greater the variation from patient to patient with respect to the characteristic being measured, the more difficult it is to be confident that the observed differences (or lack of difference) between groups is not because of this variation, rather than a true difference in treatment effects. In other words, the larger the variation among patients, the lower the statistical power.

In designing a study, the investigator chooses the size of treatment effect that is clinically important and the Type I and Type II errors he or she will accept. It is possible to design studies that maximize power for a given sample size—e.g., by choosing patients with a high event rate or similar characteristics—as long as they match the research question. But for a given data set and question the investigator cannot control the way that the characteristics of the data determine statistical power.

INTERRELATIONSHIPS

The interrelationships among the four variables discussed above are summarized in Table 9.2. The variables can be traded off against each other. In general, for any given number of patients in the study there is a trade-off between α and β error. Everything else being equal, the more

Table 9.2
Determinants of Sample Size

	Determined by		
	Investigator		The Data
N varies according to	$\dfrac{1}{\Delta, P_\alpha, P_\beta}$	and	$\dfrac{V}{I}$ or $\dfrac{I}{P}$

Where n = number of patients studied; Δ = size of difference in outcome between groups; P_α = probability of an α (Type I) error, i.e., false-positive results; P_β = probability of a β (Type II) error, i.e., false-negative result; V = variability of observations (for interval data); and P = proportion of patients experiencing outcome of interest (for nominal data) one is willing to accept one kind of error, the less it will be necessary to risk the other. Neither kind of error is inherently worse than the other. The consequences of accepting erroneous information depend on the clinical situation. When a better treatment is badly needed (e.g., when the disease is very dangerous and no satisfactory alternative treatment is available) and the proposed treatment is not dangerous, it would be reasonable to accept a relatively high risk of concluding a new treatment is effective when it really is not (large α error) to minimize the possibility of missing a valuable treatment (small β error). On the other hand, if the disease is less serious, alternative treatments are available, or the new treatment is expensive or dangerous, one might want to minimize the risk of accepting the new treatment when it is not really effective (low α error), even at the expense of a relatively large chance of missing an effective treatment (large β error). It is of course possible to reduce both α and β errors if the number of patients is increased, outcome events are more frequent, variability is decreased, or a larger treatment effect is sought.

For conventional levels of p_α and p_β, the relationship between the size of the treatment effect and the number of patients needed for a trial is illustrated by the following examples, one representing a situation in which a relatively small number of patients was sufficient and the other in which a very large number of patients was required.

> *Example* Small sample size: Case series suggest that the nonsteroidal antiinflammatory drug sulindac is active against colonic polyps. This possibility was tested in a randomized trial (6). A total of 22 patients with familial adenomatous polyposis were randomized; 11 received sulindac and 11 placebo. After 9 months, patients receiving sulindac had an average of 44% fewer polyps than those receiving placebo. This difference was statistically significant ($p = 0.014$). Because of the large effect size and the large number of polyps per patient (some had more than 100), few patients were needed to establish that the effect was beyond chance. (In this analysis it was necessary to assume that treatment affected polyps independently of which patient they occurred in—an unlikely, but probably not damaging, assumption.)

> *Example* Large sample size: The GUSTO trial, described above, was designed to include 41,000 patients to have a 90% chance of detecting a 15% reduction in mortality or a 1% decrease in mortality rate, whichever was larger, between the experimental and control treatments with a $p\alpha$ of 0.05, assuming the mortality rate in the control patients was at least 8% (2). The sample size had to be so large because a relatively small proportion of patients experienced the outcome event (death), the effect size was small (15%), and the investigators wanted a relatively high chance of detecting the effect if it were present (90%).

For most of the therapeutic questions encountered today, a surprisingly large number of patients is required. The value of dramatic, powerful treatments, such as insulin for diabetic ketoacidosis or surgery for appendicitis, could be established by studying a small number of patients. But such treatments come along rarely and many of them are already well established. We are left with diseases, many of them chronic and with multiple, interacting causes, for which the effects of new treatments are generally small. This places special importance on whether the size of clinical trials is adequate to distinguish real from chance effects.

Clinicians should be able to estimate the power of published studies. Toward that end, Figure 9.3 shows the relationship between sample size and treatment difference for several baseline rates for outcome events. It is apparent that studies involving fewer than 100 patients have a rather

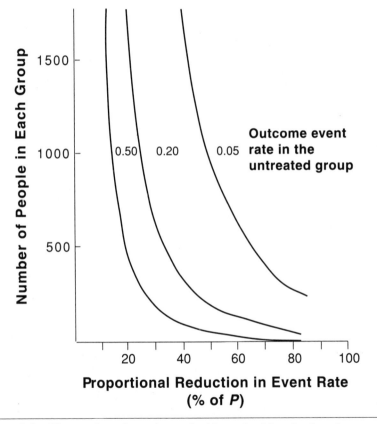

Figure 9.3. The number of people required in each of two treatment groups (of equal size) to have an 80% chance of detecting a difference ($p = 0.05$) in a given outcome rate (P) between treated and untreated patients, for various rates of outcome events in the untreated group. (Calculated from formula in Weiss NS. Clinical epidemiology. The study of the outcome of illness. New York: Oxford University Press, 1986.)

poor chance of detecting statistically significant differences of even large treatment effects. Also, it is difficult to detect effect sizes of less than 25%. In practice, statistical power can be estimated by means of readily available formulas, tables, nomograms, or computer programs.

Point Estimates and Confidence Intervals

The effect size (e.g., treatment effect in a clinical trial or relative risk in a cohort study) observed in a particular study is called the *point estimate* of the effect. It is the best estimate from the study of the true effect size and is the summary statistic usually given the most emphasis in reports of research.

However, the true effect size is unlikely to be exactly that observed in the study. Because of random variation, any one study is likely to find a result higher or lower than the true value. Therefore, a summary measure of the extent of variation that might be expected by chance is needed.

The statistical precision (stability of the estimate) of an observed effect size is expressed as a *confidence interval*, usually the 95% confidence interval, around the point estimate. Confidence intervals around an effect size are interpreted in the following manner: if the study is unbiased, there is a 95% chance that the interval includes the true effect size. The narrower the confidence interval, the more certain one can be about the size of the true effect. The true value is most likely to be close to the point estimate, less likely to be near the outer limits of the interval, and could (5 times out of 100) fall outside these limits altogether. Statistical precision increases with the statistical power of the study.

Confidence intervals contain information similar to statistical significance. If the value corresponding to no effect (such as a relative risk of 1 or a treatment difference of 0) falls outside the 95% confidence intervals for the observed effect, it is likely that the results are statistically significant at the 0.05 level. If the confidence intervals include this point, the results are not statistically significant.

But confidence intervals have other advantages. They put the emphasis where it belongs, on the size of the effect. Confidence intervals allow the reader to see the range of plausible values and so to decide whether an effect size they regard as clinically meaningful is consistent with or ruled out by the data (7). They also provide information about statistical power; if the confidence interval barely includes the value corresponding to no effect and is relatively wide, a significant difference might have been found if the study had had more power.

> *Example*   Figure 9.4 illustrates point estimates and confidence intervals for the estimated relative risk of exogenous estrogens for three diseases: endometrial cancer, breast cancer, and hip fracture. (Notice that the risk is on a log scale, giving the superficial impression that confidence intervals for

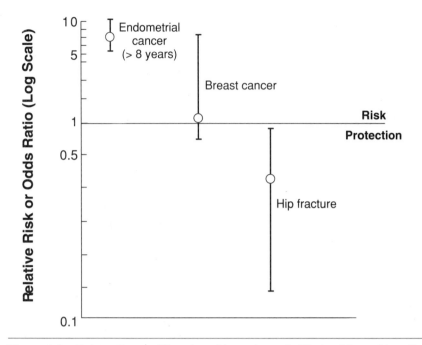

Figure 9.4.   Point estimates (O) and confidence intervals (I): the risks and benefits of exogenous estrogens for postmenopausal women. (Data from Grady D, Rubin SM, Petitti DB, Fox GS, Black D, Ettinger B, Ernster VL, Cummings SR. Hormonal therapy to prevent disease and prolong life in postmenopausal women. Ann Intern Med 1992;117:1016–1037; Colditz GA, Stampfer MJ, Willett WC, Hennekens CH, Rosner B, Speizer FE. Prospective study of estrogen replacement therapy and risk of breast cancer in postmenopausal women. JAMA 1990;264:2648–2653; and Paganini-Hill A, Ross RK, Gerkins VR, Henderson BE, Arthur M, Mack TM. Menopausal estrogen therapy and hip fractures. Ann Intern Med 1981;95:28–31.)

the higher risks are narrower than they really are.) The estimate of risk for endometrial cancer (after 8 or more years of estrogens) is 8.22, but the true value is not precisely estimated and could easily be as high as 10.61 or as low as 6.25. In any case, it is unlikely to be as low as 1.0 (no risk). In contrast, this one study suggests that estrogens are unlikely to be a risk factor for breast cancer; the best estimate of relative risk is nearly 1.0, although the data are consistent with either a small harmful or a small protective effect. Finally, estrogens are likely to protect against hip fracture. That the upper boundary of the confidence interval falls below 1.0 is another way of indicating that the protective effect is statistically significant at the 0.05 level.

Point estimates and confidence intervals are used to characterize the statistical precision of any rate (incidence and prevalence), comparisons of rates (relative and attributable risks), and other summary statistics. For example, individual studies have shown that 34% of U.S. adults have used unconventional therapy (95% confidence interval 31–37%) (8), that intensive treatment of insulin-dependent diabetes lowers the risk of development of retinopathy by 76% (95% confidence interval 62–85%) relative to conventional therapy (9), and that the sensitivity of clinical examination for splenomegaly is 27% (95% confidence interval 19–36%) (10).

Confidence intervals have become the usual way of reporting the main results of clinical research because of their many advantages over the hypothesis testing (*p* value) approach. The *p* values are still used because of tradition and as a convenience when many results are reported and it would not be feasible to include confidence intervals for all.

Statistical Power before and after a Study Is Done

Calculation of statistical power based on the hypothesis testing approach is done by the researchers before a study is undertaken to ensure that enough patients will be entered to have a good chance of detecting a clinically meaningful effect if it is present. However, after the study is completed this approach is no longer as relevant (11). There is no need to estimate effect size, outcome event rates, and variability among patients; they are now known.

Therefore, for researchers who report the results of clinical research and readers who try to understand their meaning, the confidence interval approach is more relevant. One's attention should shift from statistical power for a somewhat arbitrarily chosen effect size, which may be relevant in the planning stage, to the actual effect size observed in the study and the statistical precision of that estimate of the true value.

Detecting Rare Events

It is sometimes important to detect a relatively uncommon event (e.g., 1/1000), particularly if that event is severe, such as aplastic anemia or life-threatening arrhythmia following a drug. In such circumstances, a great many people must be observed in order to have a good chance of detecting even one such event, much less to develop a relatively stable estimate of its frequency.

Figure 9.5 shows the probability of detecting an event as a function of the number of people under observation. A rule of thumb is as follows: To have a good chance of detecting a $1/x$ event one must observe $3x$ people (12). For example, to detect a 1/1000 event, one would need to observe 3000 people.

Multiple Comparisons

The statistical conclusions of research have an aura of authority that defies challenge, particularly by nonexperts. But as many skeptics have suspected, it is possible to "lie with statistics," even if unintentionally.

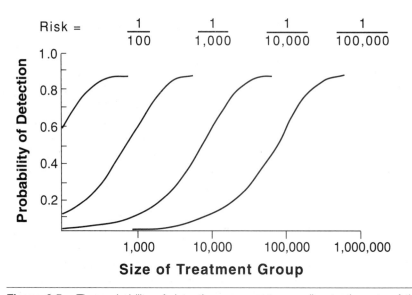

Figure 9.5. The probability of detecting one event according to the rate of the event and the number of people observed. (From Guess HA, Rudnick SA. Use of cost effectiveness analysis in planning cancer chemoprophylaxis trials. Control Clin Trials 1983; 4:89–100.)

What is more, this is possible even if the research is well designed, the mathematics flawless, and the investigators' intentions beyond reproach.

Statistical conclusions can be misleading because the strength of statistical tests depends on the number of research questions considered in the study and when those questions were asked. If many comparisons are made among the variables in a large set of data, the p value associated with each individual comparison is an underestimate of how often the result of that comparison, among the others, is likely to arise by chance. As implausible as it might seem, the interpretation of the p value from a single statistical test depends on the context in which it is done.

To understand how this might happen, consider the following example. Suppose a large study has been done in which there are multiple subgroups of patients and many different outcomes. For instance, it might be a clinical trial of the value of a treatment for coronary artery disease for which patients are in several clinically meaningful groups (e.g., 1-, 2-, and 3-vessel disease; good and bad ventricular function; the presence or absence of arrhythmias; and various combinations of these) and several outcomes are considered (e.g., death, myocardial infarction, and angina). Suppose also that there are no true associations between treatment and outcome in any of the subgroups and for any of the outcomes. Finally, suppose that the effects of treatment are assessed separately for each subgroup and for each outcome—a process that involves a great many comparisons. As pointed out earlier in this chapter, 1 in 20 of these comparisons is likely to be statistically significant at the 0.05 level. In the general case, if 20 comparisons are made, on the average, 1 would be found to be statistically significant; if 100 comparisons are made, about 5 would be likely to emerge as significant, and so on. Thus, when a great many comparisons have been made, a few will be found that are unusual enough, because of random variation, to exceed the level of statistical significance even if no true associations between variables exist in nature. The more comparisons that are made, the more likely that one of them will be found statistically significant.

This phenomenon is referred to as the *multiple comparisons* problem. Because of this problem, the strength of evidence from clinical research depends on how focused its questions were at the outset.

Unfortunately, when the results of research are presented, it is not always possible to know how many comparisons really were made. Often, interesting findings are selected from a larger number of uninteresting ones. This process of deciding what is and is not important about a mass of data can introduce considerable distortion of reality.

How can the statistical effects of multiple comparisons be taken into account when interpreting research? Although ways of adjusting p_α have been proposed, probably the best advice is to be aware of the problem and to be cautious about accepting positive conclusions of studies where multiple comparisons were made. As one statistician (13) put it:

> If you dredge the data sufficiently deeply and sufficiently often, you will find something odd. Many of these bizarre findings will be due to chance. I do not imply that data dredging is not an occupation for honorable persons, but rather that discoveries that were not initially postulated as among the major objectives of the trial should be treated with extreme caution. Statistical theory may in due course show us how to allow for such incidental findings. At present, I think the best attitude to adopt is caution, coupled with an attempt to confirm or refute the findings by further studies.

An approach to assessing the validity of statistically significant findings in subgroups was presented in Chapter 7.

Describing Associations

Statistics are also used to describe the degree of association between variables, e.g., the relationship between body mass and blood pressure. Familiar expressions of association are Pearson's product moment correlation (r) for interval data and Spearman's rank correlation for ordinal data. Each of these statistics expresses in quantitative terms the extent to which the value of one variable is associated with the value of another. Each has a corresponding statistical test to assess whether the observed association is greater than might have arisen by chance alone.

Multivariable Methods

Most clinical outcomes are the result of many variables acting together in complex ways. For example, coronary heart disease is the joint result of lipid abnormalities, hypertension, cigarette smoking, family history, diabetes, exercise, and perhaps personality. It is appropriate first to try to understand these relationships by examining relatively simple arrangements of the data, such as 2-by-2 tables (for one variable at a time) or contingency tables (stratified analyses, examining whether the effect of one variable is changed by the presence or absence of one or more other variables), because it is easy to understand the data when they are displayed in this way. However, it is usually not possible to account for more than a few variables using this method, because there are not enough patients with each combination of characteristics to allow stable estimates of rates. For example, if 120 patients were studied, 60 in each treatment group, and just one additional dichotomous variables were taken into account, there would only be at most about 15 patients in each subgroup; if patients were unevenly divided, there would be fewer in some.

What is needed then, in addition to contingency tables, is a way of examining the effects of several variables at a time. This is accomplished by *multivariable modeling,* developing a mathematical expression of the effects of many variables taken together. It is "multivariable" because it examines the effects of multiple variables simultaneously. It is "modeling" because it is a mathematical construct, calculated from the data but also based on simplifying assumptions about characteristics of the data (e.g., that the variables are all normally distributed and have the same variance).

Mathematical models can be used in studies of cause, when one wants to define the independent effect of one variable by adjusting for the effects of several other, extraneous variables. They can also be used to give more precise predictions than individual variables allow by including several variables together in a predictive model.

The basic structure of a multivariable model is

$$\text{Outcome variable} = \text{constant} + (\beta_1 \times \text{variable}_1) + (\beta_2 \times \text{variable}_2) + \ldots$$

where $\beta_1, \beta_2, \ldots$ are coefficients that are determined by the data; and variable$_1$, variable$_2$, . . . are the predictor variables that might be related to outcome. The best estimates of the coefficients are determined mathematically, depending on the powerful calculating ability of modern computers.

Modeling involves several steps.

- Identify and measure all the variables that might be related to the outcome of interest.
- Reduce the number of variables to be considered in the model to a manageable number, usually no more than several. Often this is done by selecting variables that are, when taken one at a time, most strongly related to outcome. If a statistical criterion is used at this stage, it is usual to err on the side of including variables, e.g., by choosing all variables showing an association with the outcome of interest at a cutoff level of $p < 0.10$. Evidence for the biologic importance of the variable is also considered in making the selection.
- Some variables may be strongly related to each other. If so, only one is included since both contain about the same information.
- The remaining variables are entered in the model, with the strategy for the order in which they are tried determined by the research question. For example, if some are to be controlled for in a causal analysis, they are entered in the model first, followed by the variable of primary interest. The model will then identify the independent effect of the main variable. On the other hand, if the investigator wants to make a prediction based on several variables, the variables can be entered in order of the strength of their association to the outcome variable, as determined by the model.

Modeling is now a regular feature of the medical literature, appearing in about 18% of articles in major journals (14) and in nearly all large studies of cause. Some commonly used kinds of the models are logistic regression (for dichotomous outcome variables such as occur in case-control studies) and Cox proportional hazards models (for time-to-event studies).

Multivariable modeling is an essential part of many clinical studies; there is no other way to adjust for or to include many variables at the same time. However, this advantage comes at a price. Models tend to be black boxes, and it is difficult to "get inside" them and understand how they work. Their validity is based on assumptions about the data that may not be met. They are clumsy at recognizing effect modification (different effects in different subgroups of patients). An exposure variable may be strongly related to outcome yet not appear in the model because it occurs rarely—and there is little direct information on the statistical power of the model for that variable. Finally, model results are easily affected by quirks in the data, the results of random variation in the characteristics of patients from sample to sample. It has been shown, for example, that a model frequently identified a different set of predictor variables and produced a different ordering of variables on different random samples of the same data set (15). To protect against this possibility, a rule of thumb is that there should be at least 10 outcome events for each predictor variable in the model.

For these reasons, the models themselves cannot be taken as a standard of validity; they must be independently validated. Commonly, this is done by seeing if the model predicts what is found in another, independent sample of patients (see Chapter 12). The results of the first model are considered a hypothesis, to be tested by new data. If random variation is mainly responsible for the results of the first model, it is unlikely that the same random effects will occur in the validating data set too. Other evidence for the validity of a model is its biologic plausibility and its consistency with simpler, more transparent analyses of the data such as stratified analyses.

Summary

Clinical information is based on observations made on samples of patients. Even samples that are selected without bias may misrepresent events in a larger population of such patients because of random variation in its members.

Two general approaches to assessing the role of chance in clinical observations are hypothesis testing and estimation. With the hypothesis testing approach, statistical tests are used to estimate the probability that the observed result was by chance. When two treatments are compared, there are two ways in which the conclusions of the trial can be wrong: The treatments may be no different, and it is concluded one is better; or one treatment may be better, and it is concluded there is no difference. The probabilities that these errors will occur in a given situation are called p_α and p_β, respectively.

The power of a statistical test $(1 - p_\beta)$ is the probability of finding a statistically significant difference when a difference of a given size really exists. Statistical power is related to the number of patients in the trial, size of the treatment effect, p_α, and the rate of outcome events or variability of responses among patients. Everything else being equal, power can be increased by increasing the number of patients in a trial, but that is not always feasible.

Estimation involves using the data to define the range of values that is likely to include the true effect size. Point estimates (the observed effects) and confidence intervals are used. This approach has many advantages over hypothesis testing: It emphasizes effect size, not p value; indicates the range of plausible values for the effect, which the user can relate to clinically meaningful effects; and provides information about power.

Individual studies run an increased risk of reporting a false-positive result if many subsets of the data are compared; they are at increased risk of a false-negative result if they lack statistical power, usually because they include too few patients or outcome events are uncommon.

Most clinical studies concern the effects of multiple interacting variables. With multivariable modeling, it is possible to take all into account simultaneously, either to control for extraneous variables in a causal study or to provide a stronger prediction than would be possible by including one variable at a time. However, these models must be interpreted with caution because their inner workings are relatively inaccessible, they are sensitive to random variation, and they are based on assumptions that may not be met.

REFERENCES

1. Johnson AF. Beneath the technological fix. Outliers and probability statements. J Chron Dis 1985;38:957–961.
2. The GUSTO Investigators. An international randomized trial comparing four thrombolytic strategies for acute myocardial infarction. New Engl J Med 1993;329:673–682.
3. Farkouh ME, Lang JD, Sackett DL. Thrombolytic agents: the science of the art of choosing the better treatment. Ann Intern Med 1994;120:886–888.
4. Raschke RA, Reilly BM, Guidry JR, Fontana JR, Srinivas S. The weight-based heparin dosing nomogram compared with a "standard care" nomogram. A randomized controlled trial. Ann Intern Med 1993;119:874–881.
5. Peto R, Pike MC, Armitage P, Breslow NE, Cox DR, Howard SV, Mantel N, McPherson K, Peto J, Smith PG. Design and analysis of randomized clinical trials requiring prolonged observation of each patient. I. Introduction and design. Br J Cancer 1976;34:585–612.
6. Giardiello FM, Hamilton SR, Krush AJ, Piantadosi S, Hylind LM, Celano P, Booker SV, Robinson CR, Offerhaus GJA. Treatment of colonic and rectal adenomas with sulindac in familial adenomatous polyposis. New Engl J Med 1993;328:1313–1316.
7. Braitman LE. Confidence intervals assess both clinical significance and statistical significance. Ann Intern Med 1991;114:515–517.
8. Eisenberg DM, Kessler RC, Foster C, Norlock FE, Calkins DR, Delbanco TL. Unconventional medicine in the United States. Prevalence, costs and patterns of use. New Engl J Med 1993;328:246–252.
9. Diabetes Control and Complications Trial Research Group. The effect of intensive treatment of diabetes on the development and progression of long-term complications in insulin-dependent diabetes mellitus. New Engl J Med 1993;329:977–986.
10. Grover SA, Barkun AN, Sackett DL. Does the patient have splenomegaly? JAMA 1993;270:2218–2221.
11. Goodman SN, Berlin JA. The use of predicted confidence intervals when planning experiments and the misuse of power when interpreting results. Ann Intern Med 1994;121:200–206.
12. Sackett DL, Haynes RB, Gent M, Taylor DW. Compliance. In: Inman WHW, ed. Monitoring for drug safety, Lancaster, UK: MTP Press, 1980.
13. Armitage P, Importance of prognostic factors in the analysis of data from clinical trials. Control Clin Trials 1981;1:347–353.
14. Concato J, Feinstein AR, Holford TR. The risk of determining risk with multivariable models. Ann Intern Med 1993;118:201–210.
15. Diamond GA. Future imperfect: the limitations of clinical prediction models and the limits of clinical prediction. J Am Coll Cardiol 1989;14:12A–22A.

SUGGESTED READINGS

Altman DG, Gore SM, Gardner MJ, Pocock SJ. Statistical guidelines for contributors to medical journals. Br Med J 1983;286:1489–1493.

Bailer JC III, Mosteller F, eds. Medical uses of statistics. Waltham, MA: New England Journal of Medicine Books, 1986.

Cupples LA, Heeren T, Schatzkin A, Colton T. Multiple testing of hypotheses in comparing two groups. Ann Intern Med 1984;100:122–129.

Detsky AS, Sackett DL. When was a "negative" clinical trial big enough? How many patients you need depends on what you found. Arch Intern Med 1985;145:709–712.

Facts, figures, and fallacies series

Carpenter LM. Is the study worth doing? Lancet 1993;343:221–223.

Datta M. You cannot exclude the explanation you haven't considered. Lancet 1993;342:345–347.

Glynn JR. A question of attribution. Lancet 1993;342:530–532.

Grisso JA. Making comparisons. Lancet 1993;342:157–160.

Jolley T. The glitter of the *t* table. Lancet 1993;342:27–29.

Leon D. Failed or misleading adjustment for confounding. Lancet 1993;342:479–481.

Mertens TE. Estimating the effects of misclassification. Lancet 1993;342:418–421.

Sitthi-amorn C, Poshachinda V. Bias. Lancet 1993;343:286–288.

Victoria CG. What's the denominator? Lancet 1993;342:97–99.

Friedman GD. Primer of epidemiology. 4th ed. New York: McGraw-Hill, 1994.

Gardner MJ, Altman DG. Statistics with confidence—confidence intervals and statistical guidelines. London: BMJ Books, 1989.

Goodman SN, Berlin JA. The use of predicted confidence intervals when planning experiments and the misuse of power when interpreting results. Ann Intern Med 1994;121:200–206.

Hanley JA, Lipman-Hand A. If nothing goes wrong is everything right? Interpreting zero numerators. JAMA 1983;249:1743.

Hennekens CH, Buring JE. Epidemiology in medicine. Boston: Little, Brown & Co., 1987.

Ingelfinger JA, Mosteller F, Thibodeau LA, Ware JH. Biostatistics in clinical medicine. New York: Macmillan, 1983.

Moses LE. Statistical concepts fundamental to investigations N Engl J Med 1985;312:890–897.

Riegelman RK, Hirsch RP. Studying and study and testing a test. 2nd ed. Boston: Little, Brown & Co., 1989.

Rothman KJ. A show of confidence. N Engl J Med 1978;299:1362–1363.

Young MJ, Bresnitz EA, Strom BL. Sample size nomograms for interpreting negative clinical studies. Ann Intern Med 1983;99:248–251.

10

STUDYING CASES

Each case has its lesson—a lesson which may be but is not always learned.

—Sir William Osler

Most medical knowledge has emanated from the intensive study of sick patients. The exhausted but engrossed physician at the bedside of the febrile child, chin in hand, is a favorite medical image. The presentation and discussion of a "case" is the foundation of modern medical education. Most clinicopathologic conferences and grand rounds begin with the presentation of an interesting case and then use the case to illustrate general principles and relationships. So, too, much of the medical literature is devoted to studying cases, whether narrative descriptions of a handful of cases (case reports), quantitative analyses of larger groups of patients (case series), or comparisons of groups of cases with noncases (case control studies).

Case Reports

Case reports are detailed presentations of a single case or a handful of cases. They represent an important way in which new or unfamiliar diseases, or manifestations or associations of disease are brought to the attention of the medical community. Approximately 20–30% of the original articles published in major general medical journals are studies of 10 or fewer patients.

USES OF CASE REPORTS

Case reports serve several different purposes. First, they are virtually our only means of describing rare clinical events. Therefore, they are a rich source of ideas (hypotheses) about disease presentation, risk, prognosis, and treatment. Case reports rarely can be used to test these hypotheses, but they do place issues before the medical community and often trigger more decisive studies. Some conditions that were first recognized through case reports include birth defects from thalidomide, fetal alcohol syndrome, toxic shock syndrome, Lyme disease, and HANTA virus infection.

Case reports also serve to elucidate the mechanisms of disease and treatment by reporting highly detailed and methodologically sophisticated clinical and laboratory studies of a patient or small group of patients. In this instance, the complexity, cost, and often experimental nature of the investigations limit their application to small numbers of patients. Such studies have contributed a great deal to our understanding of the genetic, metabolic, and physiologic basis of human diseases. These studies represent the bridge between laboratory research and clinical research and have a well-established place in the annals of medical progress.

The following is an example of how a report of a single case can reveal a great deal about the mechanism of a disease.

> *Example*   The anesthetic halothane was suspected of causing hepatitis. However, because the frequency of hepatitis after exposure to halothane was low and there were many other causes of hepatitis after surgery, "halothane hepatitis" was controversial.
>
> Experience with a single individual helped clarify the problem (1). An anesthetist was found to have recurrent hepatitis, leading to cirrhosis. Attacks of hepatitis regularly occurred within hours of his return to work. When he was exposed to small doses of halothane under experimental conditions, his hepatitis recurred and was well documented by clinical observations, biochemical tests, and liver histology.

Because of this unusual case, it was clear that halothane can cause hepatitis. But the case report provided no information as to whether this reaction was rare or common. Subsequent studies showed that it was not a rare reaction, which contributed to the replacement of halothane with less hepatotoxic agents.

Another use of the case report is to describe unusual manifestations of disease. Sometimes this can become the medical version of Ripley's *Believe It or Not,* an informal compendium of medical oddities, with the interest lying in the sheer unbelievability of the case. The larger the lesion and the more outrageous the foreign body, the more likely a case report is to find its way into the literature. Oddities that are simply bizarre aberrations from the usual course of events may titillate, but usually are less clinically important than other types of studies.

Some so-called oddities are, however, are the result of a fresher, more insightful look at a problem and prove to be the first evidence of a subsequently useful finding. The problem for the reader is how to distinguish between the freak and the fresh insight. There are no rules. When all else fails, one can only rely on common sense and a well-developed sense of skepticism.

BIASED REPORTING

Because case reports involve a small and highly selected group of patients, they are particularly susceptible to bias. For example, case reports of successful therapy may be misleading because journals are unlikely to receive or publish case reports of unsuccessful therapy. Perhaps the wisest stance to take when reviewing a case report is to use it as a signal to look for further evidence of the described phenomenon in the literature or among your patients.

> *Example*   A case report (2) described a 23-year-old woman who developed severe abdominal pain while on treatment with enalapril for essential hypertension. An elevated serum lipase led to a diagnosis of pancreatitis. Symptoms resolved, and the lipase returned to normal shortly after discontinuing the drug. The investigators found only one published case and began an exhaustive search of the published and unpublished literature. The search revealed an additional 60 cases, the majority of which were unpublished cases reported to the drug manufacturer. The additional cases lent strength to the possibility of a causal association between enalapril treatment and pancreatitis.

With very few exceptions, case reports on their own should not serve as the basis for altering clinical practice because of their inability to estimate the frequency of the described occurrence or the role of bias or chance.

THE JOINT OCCURRENCE OF RARE EVENTS

Case reports often describe the joint occurrence of uncommon events, particularly if the observed association lends itself to an interesting biologic explanation. But even rare events occur together by chance alone; simply observing this occurrence does not mean they are biologically related. As one author (3) put it, "In a large population the issue is not whether rare events occur, but whether they occur more frequently than expected by chance."

Table 10.1 illustrates how often two relatively uncommon conditions—end-stage renal failure and use of a specific nonsteroidal antiinflammatory drug—might occur together by chance alone. If there were no biologic association between the two (and, as discussed later in this chapter, there may well be such an association), then the probability that they would occur together is the product of their separate frequencies. In the United States alone, 100 cases would occur annually, more than enough to spawn several case reports.

There are also reasons why such cases might be seen in medical centers and be reported in the literature out of proportion to their frequency in the population at large. Patients with two severe diseases might be more likely to come to hospitals than those with either disease alone, simply because they are sicker. It has also been shown that two diseases not

Table 10.1
The Joint Occurrence of Two Rare Conditions: An Estimate of the Frequency and Number of Cases of Exposure to a Nonsteroidal Antiinflammatory Drug and End-Stage Renal Failure Occurring Together if the Two Were Not Biologically Related[a]

Frequency separately	
Prevalence of use of the drug (hypothetical)	1/100 persons
Incidence of end-stage renal disease	40/1,000,000/year
Incidence of joint occurrence	1/100 × 40/1,000,000/year
	= 4/10,000,000/year
Population of the United States	250,000,000
Cases in the United States	4/10,000,000/year × 250,000,000
	= 100/year

[a] Data from Hiatt RA, Friedman GD. Characteristics of patients referred for treatment of end-stage renal disease in a defined population. Am J Public Health 1982;72:829–833.

associated in the general population can be associated in hospitals if patients with two diseases are admitted at different rates (4). Moreover, patients with two diseases are more interesting and so are more likely to be written up in articles, submitted to journals, and accepted for publication.

Therefore, one should be skeptical about reports of association that are based on case reports only. They are simply hypotheses to be tested by stronger methods before being believed.

Case Series

A *case series* is a study of a larger group of patients (e.g., 10 or more) with a particular disease. The larger number of cases allows the investigator to assess the play of chance, and *p* values and other statistics often appear in case series, unlike in case reports. A case series is a particularly common way of delineating the clinical picture of a disease and serves this purpose well—but with important limitations.

Case series suffer from the absence of a comparison group. Occasionally, this is not a major problem.

> *Example* Between June 1981 and February 1983, a few years after AIDS was first recognized and while its manifestations were being defined, researchers from the Centers for Disease Control gathered information on 1000 patients living in the United States who met a surveillance definition for the disease. They described demographic and behavioral characteristics of patients and complications of the disease.
> *Pneumocystis carinii pneumonia* (PCP) was found in 50%, Kaposi's sarcoma in 28%, and both in 8% of patients; 14% had opportunistic infections other than PCP. All but 6% of the patients could be classified into one or more of the following groups: homosexual or bisexual men, intravenous drug abusers, Haitian natives, and patients with hemophilia (5).

This report includes no comparison group of people without AIDS. Also, the definition of cases excluded some patients who have AIDS by later standards. Nevertheless, because the complications are so uncommon in otherwise well people and the pattern of at risk groups so striking, the report clarified our view of AIDS and set the stage for more detailed studies of its manifestations and risk factors.

On the other hand, often a relatively frequent association and the absence of a comparison group have led to erroneous conclusions.

> *Example* Many physicians attribute low back pain to protrusion of one or more intervertebral disks. Several case series used magnetic resonance imaging (MRI) to define the anatomy of the lumbosacral spine in patients with low back pain. These studies found that the majority of patients had disk abnormalities, providing apparent support for the importance of disk abnormalities in low back pain. However, as described in Chapter 3, MRI studies of asymptomatic individuals revealed similar prevalences of disk abnormalities, undermining the argument that protruding disks seen on MRI are the cause of back pain (6).

Another limitation of case series is that they generally describe the clinical manifestations of disease and its treatments in a group of patients assembled at one point in time, a survival cohort (see Chapter 6). They must be distinguished, therefore, from cohort studies or trials of treatment for which an inception cohort of patients with a disease is followed over time with the purpose of looking for the outcomes of the disease. Case series often look backward in time and that restricts their value as a means of studying prognosis or cause-and-effect relationships.

Case-Control Studies

To find out whether a finding or possible cause really is more common in patients with a given disease, one needs a study with several features. First and foremost, in addition to a series of cases there must be a comparison group that does not have the disease. Second, there must be enough people in the study so that chance is less likely to play a large part in the observed results. Third, the groups must be similar enough, even though one is nondiseased, to produce a credible comparison. Finally, if one wants to show that a risk factor is independent of others—and, therefore, a possible cause—it is necessary to control for all other important differences in the analysis of the findings.

Case reports and case series cannot take us this far. Neither can cohort studies in many situations, because it is not feasible to accrue enough cases to rule out the play of chance. Case-control studies, studies that compare the frequency of a purported risk factor (generally called the "exposure") in a group of cases and a group of controls, have these features.

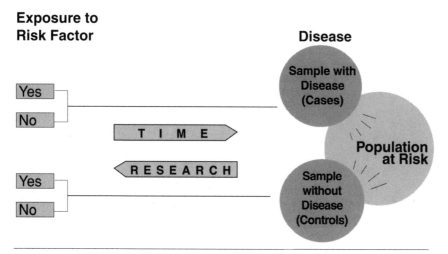

Figure 10.1. The design of case-control studies.

DESIGN

The basic design of a case-control study is diagrammed in Figure 10.1. Patients who have the disease and a group of otherwise similar people who do not have the disease are selected. The researchers then look backward in time to determine the frequency of exposure in the two groups. These data can be used to estimate the relative risk of disease related to the characteristic of interest.

> *Example* Does the use of nonsteriodal antiinflammatory drugs (NSAIDs) increase the risk of renal disease? Researchers have addressed this question using a case-control study (7). How did they go about it?
>
> First, they had to define renal disease and find a sizable group of cases available to be interviewed. For obvious reasons, they looked in tertiary care hospitals, where many such cases are gathered. The cases, of course, included only patients in whom the diagnosis had been made in the course of usual medical care. For example, asymptomatic patients with mild renal failure were much less likely to be included among the cases.
>
> Once the cases were assembled and the diagnosis confirmed, a comparison, or control,[1] group was selected. Before deciding which people to choose as controls, the investigators considered the purpose of the study. They wanted to ascertain whether patients with renal failure were more likely to have received NSAID therapy in the past than a similar group of people with no evidence of renal disease.
>
> The investigators found that the estimated relative risk of NSAID exposure for renal failure was 2.1, using data on the rates of exposure in cases and controls, and that the excess risk was largely confined to older men.

---

[1] For other uses of the word *control*, see page 129.

What is meant by *similar*? There is some controversy about this. In a cohort study of the risk of NSAIDs for renal disease, similarity would mean membership in the cohort from which the cases arose, all of whom were initially free of renal disease at the inception of the study, e.g., people residing in the same community or enrolled in the same HMO. Is there a natural cohort from which a group of cases receiving care at a given tertiary care hospital can emerge?

Because of referral practices, cases assembled at hospitals and other treatment centers usually reside in many communities, receive their care from many physicians, and belong to no common group before becoming ill. Therefore, there was no obviously similar group of people without renal disease, and one had to be created.

This was done by randomly sampling people who resided in the vicinity of each hospital. In this way, controls were assembled who, it was hoped, would provide an accurate estimate of the likely prevalence of NSAID use among the cases if there were no association between renal disease and the use of the drugs (8).

Once the cases and controls were selected and their consent obtained, the next step was to measure exposure to the risk factor of interest. The drug-taking history of each case and each control had to be reconstructed. As opposed to a cohort study where drug taking can be tracked over time, assessment of drug exposure in this case-control study relied on memory.

It is often the past that is important in case-control studies, and therein lies a potential for bias. It is difficult not to interpret the past in the light of one's present condition. For cases, this is particularly so when the present includes a disease as serious as renal failure. Investigators can attempt to avoid bias by using objective data such as computerized pharmacy records, blinding subjects to the purpose of the study, blinding observers to case status if possible, and by using carefully defined criteria to decide which of the cases and controls received prior NSAID therapy.

COHORT VERSUS CASE-CONTROL RESEARCH

Cohort and case-control studies are both observational studies of risk factors. Sometimes the two are confused. A distinguishing feature of the case-control design is that cases have the outcome of interest at the time that information on risk factors is sought. In cohort research, on the other hand, people are free of disease at the beginning of observation when the measurement of the risk factors is made. Figure 10.2 summarizes the differences between case-control and cohort designs. Since the temporal relationship between putative cause and effect is an important criterion for causality (see Chapter 11), cohort studies provide a stronger basis for a causal interpretation.

Table 10.2 summarizes the essential characteristics of cohort, case-

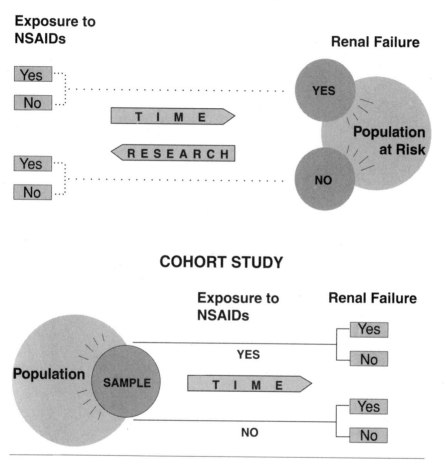

Figure 10.2   A comparison of case-control and cohort studies. Studies of NSAIDs as a risk factor for renal failure.

control, and prevalence research designs and illustrates their differences. As will be discussed later, it is these differences that make the case-control study particularly susceptible to bias.

THE ODDS RATIO

How do we decide whether there is an increased risk? Figure 10.3 shows the calculation of risk for cohort and case-control studies. In a cohort study, the susceptible population is divided into two groups—exposed to NSAIDs (A + B) and unexposed (C + D)—at the outset. Cases of renal disease emerge naturally over time in the exposed group (A) and the

Table 10.2
Summary of Characteristics of Cohort, Case-Control, and Prevalence Designs

Cohort	Case-Control	Prevalence
Begins with a defined population at risk	Population at risk often undefined	Begins with a defined population
Cases not selected but ascertained by continuous surveillance (presumably all cases)	Cases selected by investigator from an available pool of patients	Cases not selected but ascertained by a single examination of the population
Controls, the comparison group (i.e., noncases), not selected—evolve naturally	Controls selected by investigator to resemble cases	Noncases include those free of disease at the single examination
Exposure measured before the development of disease	Exposure measured, reconstructed, or recollected after development of disease	Exposure measured, reconstructed, or recollected after development of disease
Risk or incidence of disease and relative risk measured directly	Risk or incidence of disease cannot be measured directly: relative risk of exposure can be estimated by the odds ratio	Risk or incidence of disease cannot be measured directly: relative risk of exposure can be estimated by the odds ratio

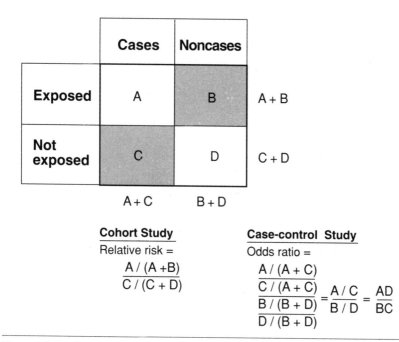

Figure 10.3 Calculation of relative risk for a cohort study and odds ratio (estimated relative risk) for a case-control study.

unexposed group (C). This provides us with appropriate numerators and denominators to calculate the incidences of renal disease in the exposed [A/(A + B)] and unexposed [C/(C + D)] cohorts. It is also possible to calculate the relative risk.

$$\text{Relative risk} = \frac{\text{Incidence of disease in the exposed}}{\text{Incidence of disease in the unexposed}} = \frac{A/(A + B)}{C/(C + D)}$$

Case-control studies, on the other hand, begin with the selection of a group of cases of renal disease (A + C) and another group of controls (B + D). There is no way of knowing disease rates because these groups are determined not by nature but by the investigators' selection criteria. Therefore, an incidence rate of disease among those exposed to NSAIDs and those not exposed cannot be computed. Consequently, it is not possible to obtain a relative risk by dividing incidence among users by incidence among nonusers. What does have meaning, however, are the relative frequencies of people exposed to NSAIDs among the cases and controls.

It has been demonstrated that one approach for comparing the frequency of exposure among cases and controls provides a measure of risk that is conceptually and mathematically similar to the relative risk. This is the *odds ratio*, defined as the odds[2] that a case is exposed divided by the odds that a control is exposed

$$\frac{[A/(A + C) \div C/(A + C)]}{[B/(B + D) \div D/(B + D)]}$$

The odds ratio simplifies to

$$\frac{A/C}{B/D} \quad \text{or} \quad \frac{AD}{BC}$$

As is seen in Figure 10.3, the odds ratio can be obtained by multiplying diagonally across the table and then dividing these cross-products.

Note that if the frequency of exposure is higher among cases, the odds ratio will exceed 1, indicating increased risk. Thus the stronger the association between the exposure and disease, the higher the odds ratio. Conversely, if the frequency of exposure is lower among cases, the odds ratio will be less than 1, indicating protection. The meaning of the odds ratio, therefore, is analogous to the relative risk obtained from cohort studies. The similarity of the information conveyed by the odds ratio and the relative risk has led some investigators to report odds ratios as "estimated relative risks" or simply "relative risks."

The odds ratio is approximately equal to the relative risk only when the incidence of disease is low, because of assumptions that must be made in the calculations. How low must the rates be? The answer depends in part on the size of the relative risk (9). In general, however, distortion of the relative risk becomes large enough to matter at disease rates in unexposed people of greater than about 1/100. Fortunately, most diseases, particularly those examined by means of case-control studies, are considerably less common than that rate.

ADVANTAGES OF CASE-CONTROL STUDIES

The case-control design has become a common and important method used to study etiology and clinical questions. What are its advantages? First, the investigators can identify cases unconstrained by the natural frequency of disease and yet can still make a comparison. Cohort studies are quite inefficient for this purpose. For example, to gather information about the risk of NSAID use in 100 individuals with end-stage renal disease, one would have to follow a cohort of 1,000,000 for about $2\frac{1}{2}$ years (see Table 10.1). Obviously, because of the expense and logistic difficulties of such a study, it would usually not be feasible. In contrast, it has been relatively inexpensive and easy to assemble 100 or more cases from hospi-

---

[2] For a reminder of what *odds* means, see page 64.

tals and other treatment facilities, find similar groups without the disease, and compare frequencies of past NSAID use. In this way, several hundred study subjects can be interviewed in a matter of weeks or months, and an answer can be obtained at a fraction of the cost of a cohort study.

A real advantage of the case-control study in exploring the effect of some causal or prognostic factors is that one need not wait for a long time for the answer. Many diseases have a long latency—the period of time between exposure to a risk factor and the expression of its pathologic effects. For example, it has been estimated that at least 10–20 years must pass before the carcinogenicity of various chemicals becomes manifest. It would require an extremely patient investigator and scientific community to wait so many years to see if a suspected risk to health can be confirmed.

Because of their ability to address important questions rapidly and efficiently, case-control studies play an increasingly prominent role in the medical literature. If one wants to study cause and effect using a relatively strong method, the case-control approach is the only practical way to study some diseases. Case-control studies comprise a growing percentage of all original articles and the majority of epidemiologic articles. Their quickness and cheapness justify their popularity as long as their results are valid; and here is the problem, because case-control studies are particularly prone to biased results. These biases are discussed in the next section.

Avoiding Bias in Case-Control Studies

In many case-control studies, the investigators create the comparison groups rather than allow nature to determine who in a population becomes a case and who remains a noncase or control as in cohort or prevalence studies. This element of manipulation is a necessary evil because the validity of a case-control study depends on the comparability of cases and controls.

Cases and controls are comparable if the controls would have been captured as cases if they developed the condition under study. In other words, to be comparable, cases and controls must be members of the same base population. A second, more controversial issue is whether to be comparable, cases and controls must have an equal opportunity to receive the exposure (10). For example, the opportunity to have received NSAIDs (discussed earlier) would presumably be greater among those who have received regular medical care and perhaps still greater among those with joint symptoms. Should both cases and controls have similar symptoms and medical care experiences. Opinions differ, but it is clear that if one insists that cases and controls have the same degree of arthritic symptoms and the same doctor, the opportunity to evaluate risk may be impossible if the doctors involved tend to either prescribe or not prescribe NSAIDs to most of their patients with common causes of musculoskeletal pain.

Therefore, ensuring comparability between cases and controls requires careful consideration of the circumstances under which an individual becomes exposed.

SELECTING CASES

In the past, most case groups in case-control studies were assembled from among patients receiving care in hospitals or other medical treatment facilities. The proliferation of disease registries, such as the National Cancer Institute's Cancer Surveillance System, and computerized diagnostic data from health plans has made it much more feasible to select all or a representative sample of all cases occurring in a defined population. Population-based cases should be more typical and include a wider spectrum of disease severity.

The cases in case-control research should, if possible, be new (incident) cases, not existing (prevalent) ones. The reasons are based on the concepts discussed in Chapter 4. The prevalence of a disease at a point in time is a function of both the incidence and duration of that disease. Duration is in turn determined by the rate at which patients leave the disease state (because of recovery or death) or persist in it because of a slow course or successful palliation. It follows from these relationships that risk factors for prevalent disease may be risk factors for either incidence and duration or both; the relative contributions of the two cannot be distinguished. An exposure that causes a particularly lethal form of the disease, thereby lowering the proportion of prevalent cases that are exposed, would result in a lowered relative risk if prevalent cases were studied. The reader can be somewhat reassured that the results of a case-control study are not biased by the selection of prevalent cases if the odds ratios obtained are similar in short- and long-duration cases.

SELECTING CONTROLS

A major potential for bias exists in many case-control studies because the controls are not a naturally occurring group, but one constructed for the study by the investigators. Which controls are appropriate in relation to the cases?

There are several strategies for choosing the right controls. First, the best way to minimize selection bias is by selecting both cases and controls from the same defined population. If cases comprise all cases or an unbiased sample of all cases arising in the population, whether accrued in a cohort study or identified in a prevalence survey, then controls can be a random sample of all the other people in the same population. This strategy is called a *population-based or nested* (in a cohort) *case-control study*. Controls should meet the same general inclusion/exclusion criteria as the cases and be sampled from the population or cohort at about the same times as the cases arose.

Example Does habitual, vigorous physical activity protect against primary cardiac arrest in people without apparent heart disease? An emergency medical information system facilitated the conduct of a population-based case-control study to answer this question (11). Cases were selected from 1250 people living in Seattle and suburban King County, Washington, who had suffered out-of-hospital primary cardiac arrest (PCA) during a defined period of time. Cases were chosen from paramedic reports; paramedics attended nearly all instances of PCA in the area at the time.

Controls were selected by dialing randomly selected telephone numbers in the same area; most people in the area had telephones in their homes. Both cases and controls had to meet criteria for entry: age 25–75 years; no clinically recognizable heart disease; no prior disease that limited activity; and a spouse who could provide information about habitual exercise, the exposure of interest. Controls were matched to cases on age, sex, marital status, and urban or suburban residence. Spouses of both cases and controls were asked about leisure-time activity. The entry criteria sought to ensure that cases and controls were members of the same base population and had opportunities to engage in physical activity.

The results, based on 163 eligible cases and controls, confirmed previous studies. The risk of PCA was 65–75% lower in persons with high-intensity leisure-time activity than in more sedentary people.

Although selecting cases and controls from a defined population or cohort is preferable, selecting both from hospitals or other health organizations is often more feasible. But studying people in health care settings is also more fallible because patients are usually a biased sample of all people in the community, the people to whom the results should apply.

A second set of strategies for having controls who are comparable to cases include the ones illustrated by the examples in this chapter and presented in Chapter 6: restriction, matching, stratification, and adjustment. Matching poses the greatest challenges and will be discussed here.

Cases can be *matched* with controls so that for each case one or more controls are selected that possess characteristics in common with the case. Researchers commonly match for age, sex, and residence, because these are frequently related to disease. But matching often extends beyond these demographic characteristics when other factors are known to be important. Matching increases the useful information obtainable from a set of cases and controls because it reduces differences between groups in determinants of disease other than the one being considered and thereby allows for a more powerful (sensitive) test of association. But matching carries a risk. If the investigator happens to match on a factor that is itself related to the exposure under study, there is an increased chance that the matched case and control will have the same history of exposure. For example, if cases and controls were matched for the presence of arthritic symptoms, which are commonly treated with NSAIDs, more matched pairs would likely have the same history of NSAID use. This process, called *overmatch-*

ing, will bias the odds ratio toward 1 and diminish the ability of a study to detect a significantly increased or decreased odds ratio.

A third strategy is to choose more than one control group. Because of the difficulties attending the selection of truly comparable control groups, a systematic error in the odds ratio may arise for any one of them. One way to guard against this possibility is to choose more than one control group from different sources.[3] One approach used when cases are drawn from a hospital is to choose one control group from other patients in the same hospital and a second control group from the neighborhoods in which the cases live. If similar odds ratios are obtained using different control groups, this is evidence against bias, because it is unlikely that bias would affect otherwise dissimilar groups in the same direction and to the same extent. If the estimates of relative risks are different, that is a signal that one or both are biased, and an opportunity exists to investigate where the bias lies.

> *Example* In a case-control study of estrogen and endometrial cancer, cases were identified from a single teaching hospital. Two control groups were selected: one from among gynecologic admissions to the same hospital and the second from a random sample of women living in the area served by the hospital.
>
> The presence of other diseases, such as hypertension, diabetes, and gallbladder disease, was much more common among the cases and the hospital control group, presumably reflecting the various forces that lead to hospitalization. Despite these differences, the two control groups reported much less long-term estrogen use than did the cases and yielded very similar odds ratios (4.1 and 3.6).
>
> The authors (12) concluded that "this consistency of results with two very different comparison groups suggests that neither is significantly biased and that the results . . . are reasonably accurate."

Options for selecting cases and controls are summarized in Figure 10.4. If cases are all occurring in a defined population (or a representative sample of all cases), then controls should be too. This is the optimal situation. If cases are a biased sample of all cases, as they are in most hospital samples, then controls should be selected with similar biases.

MEASURING EXPOSURE

Even if selection bias can be avoided in choosing cases and controls, the investigator faces problems associated with validly measuring exposure after the disease or outcome has occurred, i.e., avoiding measurement bias. Case-control studies are prone to three forms of measurement bias

---

[3] Choosing two or more control groups per case groups is different from choosing two or more controls per case. The latter is done to increase statistical power (or precision of the estimate of relative risk). In general, using more than one control subject per case results in small but useful gains in power, but there is little useful advantage to adding more controls per case beyond three or four.

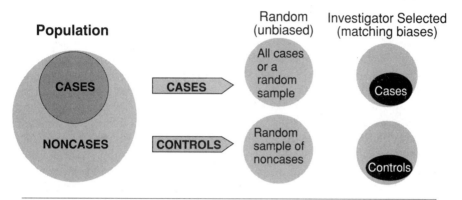

Figure 10.4   Two strategies for selecting cases and controls from the general population: unbiased samples and samples with matching biases.

because the exposure is measured after the onset of the disease or outcome under study.

1. The presence of the outcome directly affects the exposure;
2. The presence of the outcome affects the subject's recollection of the exposure; and
3. The presence of the outcome affects the measurement or recording of the exposure.

The first bias is particularly problematic if the exposure under study is a medical treatment, since the early manifestations of the illness may lead to treatment. This is sometimes referred to as confounding by indication. For example, a case-control design was used to determine whether beta-blocker drugs prevented first myocardial infarctions in patients being treated for hypertension (13). Because angina is a major indication for use of beta-blockers, the investigators carefully excluded any subjects with a history suggesting angina or other manifestation of coronary heart disease. They found that hypertensive patients treated with beta-blockers still had a significantly reduced risk of nonfatal myocardial infarctions, even after those with angina or other evidence of coronary disease were carefully excluded.

Second, people with a disease may recall exposure differently from those without the disease. With all the publicity surrounding the possible risks of various environmental exposures or drugs, it is entirely possible that victims of disease would remember their previous exposures more acutely than nonvictims or even overestimate their exposure. The influence of disease on memory status, called recall bias, must be considered when measurement of exposure relies on memory.

There are two protections against biased remembering. First, there should be alternative sources of the same information, whether written documents, such as medical or other records, or interviews with relatives or other knowledgeable individuals. Second, the specific purpose of the study should be concealed from the study subjects. It would be unethical not to inform subjects of the general nature of the study question. But to provide detailed information to subjects about the specific hypotheses could so bias the resulting information obtained as to commit another breach of ethics—involving subjects in a worthless research project.

The third problem, whether the presence of the outcome influences the way in which the exposure is measured or recorded, should be understandable to all students of physical diagnosis. If a resident admitting a patient with renal disease to the hospital is aware of a possible link between NSAID use and renal failure one could expect the resident to question the patient more intensely about previous analgesic use and to record the information more carefully. Interviewers who are aware of a possible relationship between exposure and disease and also the outcome status of the interviewee would be remarkable indeed if they conducted identical interviews for cases and controls. The protections against these sources of bias are the same as those mentioned above: multiple sources of information and blinding the data gatherers, i.e., keeping them in the dark as to the hypothesis under study.

SCIENTIFIC STANDARDS FOR CASE-CONTROL RESEARCH

It has been suggested that one should judge the validity of a case-control study by first considering how a randomized controlled trial of the same question would have been conducted (14). Of course, one could not actually do the study that way. But a randomized controlled trial would be the scientific standard against which to consider the effects of the various compromises that are inherent in a case-control study.

One would enter into a trial only those patients who could take the experimental intervention if it were offered, so in a case-control study one would select cases and controls who could have been exposed. For example, a study of whether NSAIDs are a cause of renal failure would include men and women who had no contraindications to taking NSAIDs, such as peptic ulcer. Similarly, both cases and controls should have been subjected to equal efforts to discover renal disease if it were present. These and other parallels between clinical trials and case-control studies can be exploited when trying to think through just what could go wrong, how serious a problem is it, and what can be done about it.

There have also been efforts to set out criteria for sound case-control studies (15). To apply these guidelines requires an in-depth understanding of the many possible determinants of exposure and disease, as well as the detection of both, in actual clinical situations.

USING CASE-CONTROL STUDIES TO EXAMINE HEALTH CARE

The major use of case-control studies has been to test hypotheses about the etiology of disease. More recently, investigators have exploited the advantages of the case-control design to study questions related to the provision and quality of health care.

> *Example* Is cerebral palsy and fetal death preventable? British investigators (16) used a case-control design to compare the antepartum care received by 141 babies developing cerebral palsy and 62 dying intrapartum or neonatally. Each case was matched with two healthy babies born at the same time and place. A failure to respond to signs of severe fetal distress was more common among cases than controls but only accounted for a very small percentage of babies with cerebral palsy.

Because most serious adverse effects of poor-quality medical care are relatively rare, the case-control design provides an efficient strategy for examining the relationship between deviations from guidelines or other protocols and poor outcomes.

Summary

Much of medical progress is derived from the careful study of sick individuals. Case reports are studies of just a few patients, e.g., ≤10. They are a useful means of describing unusual presentations of disease, examining the mechanisms of disease, and raising hypotheses about causes and treatments. However, case reports are particularly prone to bias and chance. Case series—studies of larger collections of patients—still suffer from the absence of a reference group with which to compare the experience of the cases and from sampling cases at various times in the course of their disease.

In case-control studies, a group of cases is compared with a similar group of noncases (controls). A major advantage resides in the ability to assemble cases from treatment centers or disease registries as opposed to finding them or waiting for them to develop in a defined population at risk. Thus case-control studies are much less expensive and much quicker to perform than cohort studies and the only feasible strategy for studying risk factors for rare diseases. Relative risk can be estimated by the odds ratio, although it is not possible to compute incidences or relative risk directly. The disadvantages of the case-control design all relate to its considerable susceptibility to bias. This problem is most related to two characteristics of case-control research. First, the groups to be compared are commonly constructed by the researcher and are not constituted naturally; second, the exposure is measured after the disease has already occurred.

Given the vulnerability of case-control studies to bias, what place do they have in clinical epidemiologic research? To some, case-control studies are unscientific, illogical, and a curse. To others, they are viewed as the essential first step in studying many medically important questions. There is nearly universal agreement that cohort studies provide stronger, more valid evidence and, if feasible, are the design of choice. But with appropriate attention to possible sources of bias, case-control studies can provide a valid and efficient method to answer many clinical and health services questions.

REFERENCES

 1. Klatskin G, Kimberg DV. Recurrent hepatitis attributable to halothane sensitization in an anesthetist. N Engl J Med 1969;280:515–522.
 2. Roush MK, McNutt RA, Gray TF. The adverse effect dilemma: quest for accessible information. Ann Intern Med 1991;114:298–299.
 3. Mulvihill JJ. Clinical ecogenetics. Cancer in families. N Engl J Med 1985;312:1569–1570.
 4. Berkson J. Limitations of the application of fourfold table analysis to hospital data. Biomed Bull 1946;2:47–53.
 5. Jaffe HW, Bregman DJ, Selik RM. Acquired immune deficiency syndrome in the United States: the first 1,000 cases. J Infect Dis 1983;148:339–345.
 6. Jensen MC, Brant-Zawadzki MN, OBuchowski N. Modic MT, Malkasian D, Ross JS. Magnetic resonance imaging of the lumbar spine in people without back pain. N Engl J Med 1994;331:69–73.
 7. Sandler DP, Burr FR, Weinberg CR. Non-aspirin nonsteroidal antiinflammatory drugs and risk of chronic renal disease. Ann Intern Med 1991;115:165–172.
 8. Schlesselman JJ. Case control studies: design, conduct, analysis. New York: Oxford University Press, 1982.
 9. Feinstein AR. The bias caused by high values of incidence for P_1 in the odds ratio assumption that $1 - P_1 \approx 1$. J Chron Dis 1986;39:485–487.
10. Wacholder S, McLaughlin JK, Silverman DT, Mandel JS. Selection of controls in case-control studies. Am J Epidemiol 1992;135:1019–1028.
11. Siscovick DS, Weiss NS, Hallstrom AP, Inui TS, Peterson DR. Physical activity and primary cardiac arrest. JAMA 1982;248:3113–3117.
12. Hulka BS, Fowler WC Jr, Kaufman DG, Greenberg BG, Hogue CJR, Berger GS, Pulliam CC. Estrogen and endometrial cancer: cases and two control groups from North Carolina. Am J Obstet Gynecol 1980;137:92–101.
13. Psaty BM, Koepsell TD, LoGerfo JP, Wagner EH, Inui TS. Beta-blockers and primary prevention of coronary heart disease in patients with high blood pressure. JAMA 1989;261:2087–2094.
14. Feinstein AR, Horwitz RI. Double standards, scientific methods and epidemiologic research. N Engl J Med 1982;307:1611–1617.
15. Horwitz R, Feinstein AR. Methodologic standards and contradictory results in case control research. Am J Med 1979;66:556–564.
16. Gaffney G. Sellers S, Flavell V, Squier M, Johnson A. Case-control study of intrapartum care, cerebral palsy, and perinatal death. Br Med J 1994;308:743–750.

SUGGESTED READINGS

Feinstein AR. Clinical biostatistics XX: the epidemiologic trohoc, the ablative risk ratio, and "retrospective research." Clin Pharmacol Ther 1973;14:291–307.

Feinstein AR, Horwitz RI, Spitzer WO, Battista RN. Coffee and pancreatic cancer: the problems of etiologic science and epidemiological case-control research. JAMA 1981;246:957–961.

Hayden GF, Kramer MS, Horwitz RI. The case-control study. A practical review for the clinician. JAMA 1982;247:326–331.

Ibrahim MA, Spitzer WO. The case-control study: consensus and controversy. New York: Pergamon Press, 1979.

Rothman KJ. Modern epidemiology. Boston: Little, Brown & Co., 1986.

11

CAUSE

Example Some years ago, medical students were presented a study of the relationship between the cigarette smoking habits of obstetricians and the vigor of babies they delivered. Infant vigor is measured by an Apgar score; a high score (9–10) indicates that the baby is healthy, whereas a low score indicates the baby might be in trouble and require close monitoring. The study suggested that smoking by obstetricians (not in the delivery suite!) had an adverse effect on Apgar scores in newborns. The medical students were then asked to comment on what was wrong with this study. After many suggestions, someone finally said that the conclusion simply did not make sense.

It was then acknowledged that, although the study was real, the "exposure" and "disease" had been altered for the presentation. Instead of comparing smoking habits of obstetricians with Apgar scores of newborns, the study, published in 1843 by Oliver Wendell Holmes (then professor of anatomy and physiology and later dean of Harvard Medical School), concerned hand washing habits by obstetricians and subsequent puerperal sepsis in mothers. The observations led Holmes (1) to conclude: "The disease known as puerperal fever is so far contagious, as to be frequently carried from patient to patient by physicians and nurses."

One mid-19th century response to Holmes's assertion that unwashed hands caused puerperal fever was remarkably similar to that of the medical students: The findings made no sense. "I prefer to attribute them [puerperal sepsis cases] to accident, or Providence, of which I can form a conception, rather than to contagion of which I cannot form any clear idea, at least as to this particular malady," wrote Dr. Charles D. Meigs, professor of midwifery and the diseases of women and children at Jefferson Medical College (1).

Holmes and Meigs were confronted with a question about cause. Holmes was convinced by his data that the spread of puerperal sepsis was caused by obstetricians not washing their hands between deliveries. He could not, however, supply the pathogenetic mechanism by which hand washing was related to the disease, as bacteria had not yet been discovered. Meigs, therefore, remained unconvinced that the cause of puerperal sepsis had been established (and presumably did not bother to wash his hands).

Clinicians frequently are confronted with information about possible causal relationships. In fact, most of this book has been about methods used to establish cause, although we have not called special attention to the term.

In this chapter, we review concepts of cause in clinical medicine. We then outline the kinds of evidence that, when present, strengthen the likelihood that an association represents a causal relationship. We also deal briefly with a kind of research design not yet considered in this book: studies in which exposure to a possible cause is known only for groups and not specifically for individuals in the groups.

Concepts of Cause

Webster's (2) defines *cause* as "something that brings about an effect or a result." In medical textbooks, cause is usually discussed under such headings as "etiology," "pathogenesis," "mechanisms," or "risk factors."

Cause is important to practicing physicians primarily in guiding their approach to three clinical tasks: prevention, diagnosis, and treatment. The clinical example at the beginning of this chapter illustrates how knowledge of cause-and-effect relationships can lead to successful preventive strategies. Likewise, when we periodically check patients' blood pressures, we are reacting to evidence that hypertension causes morbidity and mortality and that treatment of hypertension prevents strokes and myocardial infarction. The diagnostic process, especially in infectious disease, frequently involves a search for the causative agent. Less directly, the diagnostic process often depends on information about cause when the presence of risk factors is used to identify groups of patients in whom disease prevalence is high (see Chapter 3). Finally, belief in a causal relationship underlies every therapeutic maneuver in clinical medicine. Why give penicillin for pneumococcal pneumonia unless we think it will cause a cure? Or advise a patient with metastatic cancer to undergo chemotherapy unless we believe the antimetabolite will cause a regression of metastases and a prolongation of survival, comfort, and/or ability to carry on daily activities?

By and large, clinicians are more interested in treatable or reversible than immutable causes. Researchers, on the other hand, might also be interested in studying causal factors for which no efficacious treatment or prevention exists, in hopes of developing preventive or therapeutic interventions in the future.

SINGLE AND MULTIPLE CAUSES

In 1882, 40 years after the Holmes-Meigs confrontation, Koch set forth postulates for determining that an infectious agent is the cause of a disease. Basic to his approach was the assumption that a particular disease has one cause and a particular cause results in one disease. He stipulated that:

1. The organism must be present in every case of the disease;
2. The organism must be isolated and grown in pure culture;
3. The organism must cause a specific disease when inoculated into an animal; and
4. The organism must then be recovered from the animal and identified.

Interestingly, he did not consider the effect of treatment in establishing cause, something he might have added a century later when effective treatments had become more common in medicine.

Koch's postulates contributed greatly to the concept of cause in medicine. Before Koch, it was believed that many different bacteria caused any given disease. The application of his postulates helped bring order out of chaos. They are still useful today. That a given organism causes a given disease was the basis for the discovery in 1977 that Legionnaire's disease is caused by a Gram-negative bacterium, and the determination in the 1980s that the newly discovered HIV causes AIDS.

For most diseases, however, cause cannot be established simply by Koch's rules. Sometimes, too much reliance on Koch's approach has gotten the medical community into trouble by narrowing our perspectives. Would that disease was so simple that we always had a single cause–single disease relationship. Smoking causes lung cancer, chronic obstructive pulmonary disease, peptic ulcers, bladder cancer, and coronary artery disease. Coronary artery disease has multiple causes, including cigarette smoking, hypertension, hypercholesterolemia, and heredity. It is also possible to have coronary artery disease without any of these known risk factors.

Usually, many factors act together to cause disease in what has been called the "web of causation" (3). A causal web is well understood in conditions such as coronary artery disease, but is also true for infectious diseases, where presence of the organism is *necessary* for disease to occur but not necessarily *sufficient*. AIDS cannot occur without exposure to HIV, but exposure to the virus does not necessarily result in disease. For example, exposure to HIV rarely results in AIDS after needlesticks (3 or 4/1000), because the virus is not nearly as infectious as, say, the hepatitis B virus.

PROXIMITY OF CAUSE TO EFFECT

When biomedical scientists study cause, they usually search for the underlying pathogenetic mechanism or final common pathway of disease. Sickle-cell anemia is an example, with the genetic change associated with hemoglobin S (HbS) leading to polymerization and erythrocytic sickling when HbS gives up its oxygen. Elucidating pathogenesis of disease has played a crucial part in the advancement of medical science in this century.

However, disease is also determined by less specific, more remote causes, or risk factors, such as people's behavior or characteristics of their environments. These factors may be even more important causes of disease than are pathogenetic mechanisms. For example, a large proportion of cardiovascular and cancer deaths in the United States can be traced to behavioral and environmental factors; the spread of AIDS is due primarily to sexual behaviors and drug use; and deaths from violence and accidents are rooted in social conditions, access to guns, and alcohol and seatbelt use.

To view cause in medicine exclusively as cellular and subcellular processes restricts the possibilities for useful clinical interventions. If the pathogenetic mechanism is not clear, knowledge of risk factors may still lead to very effective treatments and preventions. Thus Holmes was right in his assertion that obstetricians should wash their hands, even though he had little notion of bacteria.

For many diseases, both pathogenetic mechanisms and nonspecific risk factors have been important in the spread and control of the diseases. Sometimes the many different causes interact in complicated ways.

Example   Koch's postulates were originally used to establish that tuberculosis is caused by inoculation of the acid-fast bacillus *Mycobacterium tuberculosis* into susceptible hosts. The final common pathway of tuberculosis is the invasion of host tissue by the bacteria. From a pathogenetic perspective, conquering the disease required antibiotics or vaccines that were effective against the organism. Through biomedical research efforts, both have been achieved.

However, the development of the disease tuberculosis is far more complex. Other important causes are the susceptibility of the host and the degree of exposure (Fig. 11.1). In fact, these causes determine whether invasion of host tissue can occur.

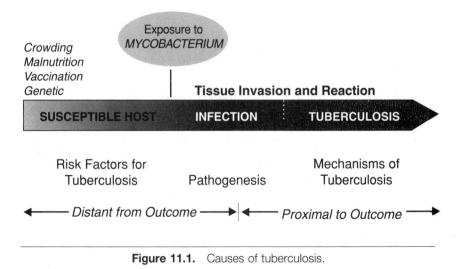

Figure 11.1.   Causes of tuberculosis.

Some clinicians would be hesitant to label host susceptibility and level of exposure as causes of tuberculosis, but they are very important components of cause. In fact, social and economic improvements influencing host susceptibility, such as less crowded living space and better nutrition, may have played a more prominent role in the decline in tuberculosis rates in developed countries than treatments developed through the biomedical-pathogenetic research model. Figure 11.2A shows that the death rate from tuberculosis had dropped dramatically long before antibiotics were introduced. (The vaccine came even later.)

Since 1985 the number of TB cases in the United States has increased (4) (Fig. 11.2B). Why is this so? A total of 60% of the increase occurred in foreign-born persons. HIV infections are also a factor, with an increasing number of susceptible people, as AIDS spreads and weakens the immune systems of its victims. These susceptible hosts are more likely than the general population to be exposed to tuberculosis, because both AIDS and tuberculosis are more common in economically depressed populations. Finally, changes have occurred in the bacillus itself, with the evolution of multidrug resistant strains. To complicate the picture further, multidrug resistance also is caused by a web of circumstances. Genetic changes in the *Mycobacterium* are more likely to occur with medication noncompliance (5), which is more likely among intravenous drug users, an important risk group for AIDS. Changes in the bacterium's genetic makeup may also be related to high replication rates in immunodeficient hosts. Thus the interplay of environment, behavior and subcellular biology may be incredibly complex when thinking about cause.

Another example of the importance of both pathogenetic and epidemiologic approaches to cause is the recent decline in deaths from coronary artery disease in the United States.

> *Example* During the past two decades, the death rate from coronary artery disease has dropped more than a third. This decline accompanied decreased exposure, in the population as a whole, to several risk factors for cardiovascular disease: A larger proportion of people with hypertension are being treated effectively, middle-aged men are smoking less, and fat and cholesterol consumption has declined. These developments were, at least in part, the result of both epidemiologic and biomedical studies and have spared tens of thousands of lives per year. It is doubtful that they would have occurred without understanding of both the proximal mechanisms and the more remote origins of cardiovascular disease (6).

INTERPLAY OF MULTIPLE CAUSES

When more than one cause act together, the resulting risk may be greater or less than would be expected by simply combining the effects of the separate causes. Clinicians call this phenomenon synergism if the joint

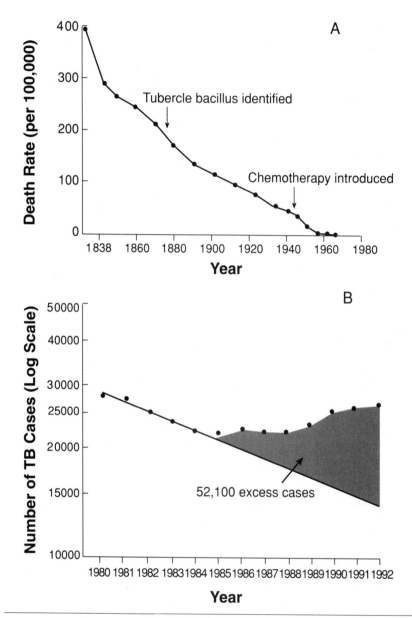

Figure 11.2.   A, Declining death rate from respiratory tuberculosis in England and Wales over the past 150 years. (From McKeown T. The role of medicine: dream, mirage or nemesis. London: Nuffield Provincial Hospital Trust, 1976.) **B,** Excess tuberculosis cases in the United States, 1985–1992. Difference between expected and observed number of cases. *Dotted line,* observed cases; *solid line,* expected cases. (From Cantwell MF, et al. Epidemiology of tuberculosis in the United States, 1985 through 1992. JAMA 1994;272:535–539.)

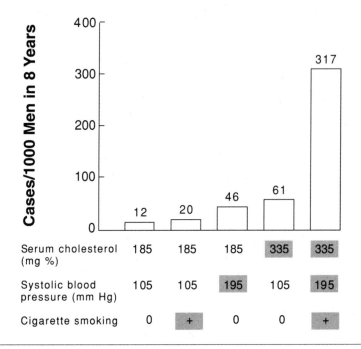

Serum cholesterol (mg %)	185	185	185	335	335
Systolic blood pressure (mm Hg)	105	105	195	105	195
Cigarette smoking	0	+	0	0	+

Figure 11.3.   Interaction of multiple causes of disease. The risk of developing cardiovascular disease in men according to the level of several risk factors alone and in combination. Abnormal values are in shaded boxes. (Redrawn from Kannel WB. Preventive cardiology. Postgrad Med 1977;61:74–85.)

effect is greater than the sum of the effects of the individual causes, and antagonism if it is less.[1]

> *Example*   Figure 11.3 shows the probability of developing cardiovascular disease over an 8-year period among men aged 40. Men who did not smoke cigarettes, had low serum cholesterol values, and had low systolic blood pressure readings were at low risk of developing disease (12/1000). Risk increased, in the range of 20 to 61/1000, when the various factors were present individually. But when all three factors were present, the absolute risk of cardiovascular disease (317/1000) was almost three times greater than the sum of the individual risks (7).

Elucidation of cause is more difficult when many factors play a part than when a single one predominates. However, when multiple causative

---

[1] *Statistical interaction* is present when combinations of variables in a mathematical model add to the model's explanatory power after the net effects of the individual predictor variables have been taken into account. It is conceptually related to biologic synergy and antagonism but is a mathematical construct, not an observable phenomenon in nature.

factors are present and interact, it may be possible to make a substantial impact on a patient's health by changing only one, or a small number, of the causes. Thus, in the previous example, getting patients to give up smoking and treating hypertension might substantially lower the risk of developing cardiovascular disease in men, even in the continuing presence of other causative factors.

EFFECT MODIFICATION

Effect modification is a special type of interaction. It is present when the strength of the relationship between two variables is different according to the level of some third variable, called an *effect modifier.*

> **Example** Because of conflicting results of studies evaluating the effectiveness of thiazide diuretics in preventing coronary heart disease, a study was done to examine whether there was a relationship between the dose of thiazide and the risk of sudden death, and whether adding potassium-sparing therapy modified the effect. Figure 11.4 summarizes the results. The dose of thiazide determines its effect, with a low dose, 25 mg, protecting against sudden death and a high dose, 100 mg, increasing the chances of sudden death. Adding potassium-sparing therapy modifies the effect at several doses, adding a protective effect (8).

Establishing Cause

In clinical medicine, it is not possible to prove causal relationships beyond any doubt. It is only possible to increase one's conviction of a cause-and-effect relationship, by means of empiric evidence, to the point at which, for all intents and purposes, cause is established. Conversely, evidence against a cause can be mounted until a cause-and-effect relationship becomes implausible. The possibility of a postulated cause-and-effect relationship should be examined in as many different ways as possible. This usually means that several studies must be done to build evidence for or against cause.

ASSOCIATION AND CAUSE

Two factors—the suspected cause and the effect—obviously must appear to be associated if they are to be considered as cause and effect. However, not all associations are causal. Figure 11.5 outlines other kinds of associations that must be excluded. First, a decision must be made as to whether an apparent association between a purported cause and an effect is real or merely an artifact because of bias or random variation. Selection and measurement biases and chance are most likely to give rise to apparent associations that do not exist in nature. If these problems can be considered unlikely, a true association exists. But before deciding that the association is causal, it is necessary to know if the association occurs indirectly, through another (confounding) fac-

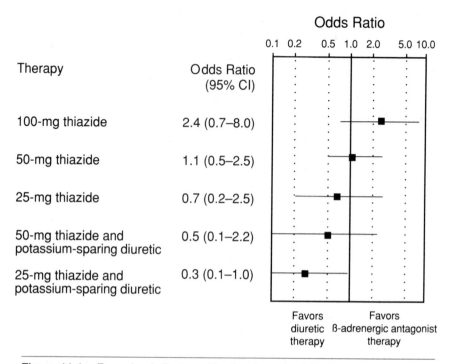

Figure 11.4. Example of effect modification: how the risk of cardiac arrest in patients using thiazide diuretics (compared with the risk of cardiac arrest in patients using beta-blockers) changes according to use of potassium-sparing diuretics. Odds ratios—with 95% confidence intervals (CI)—increase with increasing dose of diuretic, suggesting that it is safer to use beta-blockers than thiazide diuretics. However, with the addition of potassium-sparing diuretics, thiazide diuretics cause a lower risk of cardiac arrest than beta-blocker therapy. (Redrawn from Siscovick DS, et al. Diuretic therapy for hypertension and the risk of primary cardiac arrest. N Engl J Med 1994;330:1852–1857.)

tor, or directly. If confounding is not found, a causal relationship is likely.

At some future time another factor may be found that is more directly causal. For example, several studies found that women fared more poorly than men after coronary bypass surgery and it was thought that sex was related to postoperative prognosis. On further study, small body surface area—which correlated with small-diameter coronary arteries—was found to be an important variable leading to heart failure and death, not being female per se (9). Thus factors that are considered causes at one time are sometimes found to be indirectly related to disease later, when more evidence is available.

EXPLANATION	FINDING

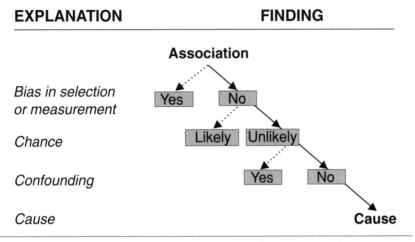

Figure 11.5.   Association and cause.

RESEARCH DESIGN

When considering a possible causal relationship, the strength of the research design used to establish the relationship is an important piece of evidence.

Of the research designs so far discussed in this book, well-conducted randomized controlled trials, with adequate numbers of patients; blinding of therapists, patients, and researchers; and carefully standardized methods of measurement and analysis are the best evidence for a cause-and-effect relationship. Randomized controlled trials guard against differences in the groups being compared, both for factors already known to be important, which can be overcome by other methods, and for unknown confounding factors.

We ordinarily use randomized controlled trials to provide evidence about causal relationships for treatments and prevention. However, as pointed out in Chapter 6, randomized controlled trials are rarely feasible when studying causes of disease. Observational studies must be used instead.

In general, the further one must depart from randomized trials, the less the research design protects against possible biases and the weaker the evidence is for a cause-and-effect relationship. Well-conducted cohort studies are the next best design, because they can be performed in a way that minimizes known confounding, selection and measurement biases. Cross-sectional studies are vulnerable because they provide no direct evidence of the sequence of events. True prevalence surveys— cross-sectional studies of a defined population—guard against selection bias but are subject to measurement and confounding biases. Case-control studies are vulnerable to selection bias as well. Weakest of all are cases series, because they have no defined population and no comparison group.

This hierarchy of research designs is only a rough guide, based on extent of susceptibility to bias. The manner in which an individual study is performed can do a great deal to increase or decrease its validity, regardless of the type of design used.

POPULATION STUDIES

Up until now, we have discussed evidence for cause when exposure and disease status are known for each individual in the study. In a different kind of research, most often used for epidemiologic studies of large populations, exposure is known only for the groups, not for the individuals in the groups.

Studies in which exposure to a risk factor is characterized by the average exposure of the group to which individuals belong are called *aggregate risk studies.* Another term is *ecological studies,* because people are classified by the general level of exposure in their environment.

> *Example* What factors are associated with cardiac mortality in developed countries? St. Leger et al. (10) gathered data on rates of ischemic heart disease mortality in 18 developed countries to explore the contribution of various economic, health services, and dietary variables. One finding that was not anticipated was a strong negative association between ischemic heart disease death and wine consumption (Fig. 11.6).
>
> This study raises the hypothesis that alcohol protects against ischemic heart disease. Since then, studies on individuals have shown that levels of serum high-density lipoprotein, a protective factor for cardiovascular disease, are increased by alcohol consumption.

Aggregate risk studies are rarely definitive in and of themselves. The main problem is a potential bias called the *ecological fallacy:* Affected individuals in a generally exposed group may not themselves have been exposed to the risk. Also, exposure may not be the only characteristic that distinguishes people in the exposed group from those in the nonexposed group, i.e., there may be confounding factors. Thus aggregate risk studies are most useful in raising hypotheses, which must then be tested with more rigorous research.

TIME SERIES STUDIES

Evidence from aggregate risk studies that a factor is actually responsible for an effect can be strengthened if observations are made at more than two points in time (before and after) and in more than one place. In a *time series study,* the effect is measured at various points in time before and after the purported cause has been introduced. It is then possible to see if the effect varies as expected. If changes in the purported cause are followed

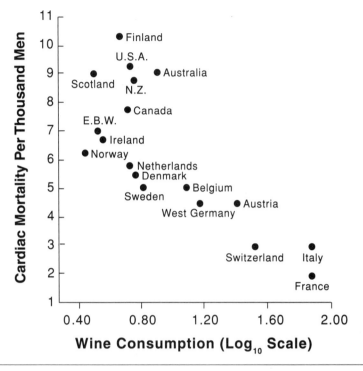

Figure 11.6.   Example of an aggregate risk study: relationship between wine consumption and cardiac mortality in developed countries. (Drawn from St. Leger AS, Cochrane AL, Moore F. Factors associated with cardiac mortality in developed countries with particular reference to the consumption of wine. Lancet 1979; 1:1017–1020.)

by changes in the purported effect, the association is less likely to be spurious.

> *Example*   The risk of *Clostridium difficile*-associated diarrhea and pseudo-membranous colitis has been shown to be related to the use of antibiotics, particularly clindamycin, ampicillin, and cephalosporins. An epidemic of *C. difficile* diarrhea broke out in a hospital in 1990 after use of clindamycin increased sharply (Fig. 11.7) (11). Education, infection control, and environmental hygiene efforts were immediately instituted, but the epidemic continued unabated. Clindamycin was then removed from the hospital formulary, and its use plummeted, along with the number of cases of *C. difficile*-diarrhea. To investigate the association further, the authors conducted a case-control study, which corroborated the findings of the time series analysis.

In a *multiple time series study*, the suspected cause is introduced into several different groups at various times. Measurements of effect are then made among the groups to determine if the effect occurs in the same sequential manner in which the suspected cause was introduced. If the effect regularly follows introduction of the suspected cause at various times and places, there is stronger evidence for cause than if this phenomenon is observed only once, because it is even more improbable that the same extraneous factor(s) occurred at the same time in relation to the cause in many different places and eras.

> *Example*   Because there were no randomized controlled trials of cervical cancer screening programs before they became widely accepted, their effectiveness must be evaluated by means of observational studies. A multiple time series study has provided some of the most convincing evidence of their effectiveness (12). Data were gathered on screening programs begun in the various Canadian provinces at various times during a 10-year period in the 1960s and 1970s. Reductions in mortality regularly followed the introduction of screening programs regardless of time and location. With these data, it

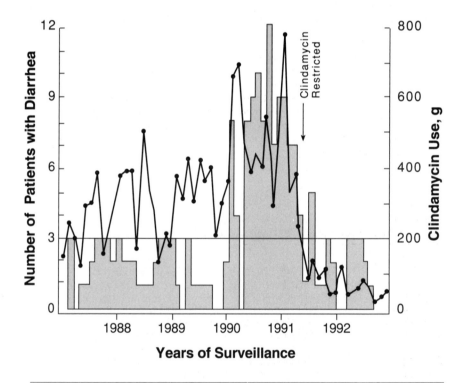

Figure 11.7.   A time-series study of the relationship of clindamycin use and *Clostridium difficile*-associated diarrhea. (Redrawn from Pear SM, Williamson TH, Bettin KM, Gerding DN, Galgiani JN. Decrease in nosocomial *Clostridium difficile*-associated diarrhea by restricting clindamycin use. Ann Intern Med 1194;120:272–277.)

was concluded that "screening had a significant effect on reduction in mortality from carcinoma of the uterus."

ELEMENTS FOR OR AGAINST CAUSE

In 1965, the British statistician Sir Austin Bradford Hill (13) proposed a set of features that should be sought when deciding whether a relationship between a sickness and some environmental factor is causal or just an association. His proposals have been widely used, sometimes with modifications (Table 11.1). We will comment briefly on the individual elements. They are not all of equal weight in deciding about cause.

Temporal Relationships between Cause and Effect

Causes should obviously precede effects. This fundamental principle seems self-evident, but it can be overlooked when interpreting most cross-sectional studies and case-control studies, in which both the purported cause and the effect are measured at the same point in time. It is sometimes assumed that one variable precedes another without actually establishing that this is so. In other cases, it may be difficult to establish which came first.

> *Example*   It has long been noted that overweight persons are at higher risk of death, especially cardiovascular death, than people with normal weight. Thus it is reasonable to assume that weight loss would be protective among overweight people. However, several cohort studies have found excess mortality among people who lose weight, even among people without any apparent preexisting disease. These distressing findings may be explained if a subtle, preclinical effect of fatal illness is weight loss (14). Thus fatal conditions may precede and cause weight loss, not vice versa. (This possibility could be excluded if it was known whether the weight loss was voluntary in those losing weight.)

Table 11.1
Evidence That an Association Is Cause and Effect[a]

Criteria	Comments
Temporality	Cause precedes effect
Strength	Large relative risk
Dose-response	Larger exposures to cause associated with higher rates of disease
Reversibility	Reduction in exposure associated with lower rates of disease
Consistency	Repeatedly observed by different persons, in different places, circumstances, and times
Biologic plausibility	Makes sense, according to biologic knowledge of the time
Specificity	One cause leads to one effect
Analogy	Cause-and-effect relationship already established for a similar exposure or disease

[a] Modified from Bradford-Hill AB. The environment and disease: association and causation. Proc R Soc Med 1965;58:295–300.

Although it is absolutely necessary for a cause to precede an effect in clinical medicine—and, therefore, the lack of such a sequence is powerful evidence against cause—an appropriate temporal sequence alone is weak evidence for cause.

Strength of the Association

A strong association between a purported cause and an effect, as expressed by a large relative or absolute risk, is better evidence for a causal relationship than a weak association. Thus the 4- to 16-fold higher incidence of lung cancer among smokers than nonsmokers in many different prospective studies is much stronger evidence that smoking causes lung cancer than the findings in these same studies that smoking may be related to renal cancer, for which the relative risks are much smaller (1.1–1.6) (15). Similarly, that the relative risk of hepatitis B infection for hepatocellular cancer is nearly 300 leaves little doubt that the virus is a cause of liver cancer (16). Bias can sometimes result in large relative risks. However, unrecognized bias is less likely to produce large relative risks than to produce small ones.

Dose-Response Relationships

A dose-response relationship is present when varying amounts of the purported cause are related to varying amounts of the effect. If a dose-response relationship can be demonstrated, it strengthens the argument for cause and effect. Figure 11.8 shows a clear dose-response curve when lung cancer death rates (responses) are plotted against number of cigarettes smoked (doses).

Although a dose-response curve is good evidence for a causal relationship, especially when coupled with a large relative or absolute risk, its existence does not exclude confounding factors.

> *Example* Both the strong association between smoking and lung cancer and the dose-response relationship have been dismissed by the tobacco industry as examples of confounding. According to this argument, there is some unknown variable that both causes people to smoke and increases their risk of developing lung cancer. The more the factor is present, the more both smoking and lung cancer are found—hence, the dose-response relationship. Such an argument is a theoretically possible explanation for the association between smoking and lung cancer, although just what the confounding factor might be has never been clarified. Short of a randomized controlled trial (which would, on the average, allocate the people with the confounding factor equally to smoking and nonsmoking groups) the confounding argument is difficult to refute completely.

Reversible Associations

A factor is more likely to be a cause of disease if its removal results in a decreased risk of disease, i.e., the association between suspected cause and effect is reversible. Figure 11.9 shows that when people give up smoking they decrease their likelihood of getting lung cancer.

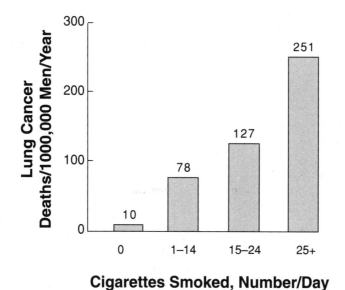

Figure 11.8. Example of a dose-response relationship: lung cancer deaths according to dose of cigarettes in male physicians. (Drawn from Doll R, Peto R. Mortality in relation to smoking: 20 years' observations on male British doctors. Br Med J 1976;2:1525–1536.)

Reversible associations are strong, but not infallible, evidence of a causal relationship. Confounding could conceivably explain a reversible association. For example, in Figure 11.9 it is possible (but unlikely) that people willing to give up smoking have smaller amounts of the unidentified factor than those who continue to smoke.

Consistency

When several studies conducted at different times in different settings and with different kinds of patients all come to the same conclusion, evidence for a causal relationship is strengthened. That screening for colorectal cancer is effective becomes more plausible when a randomized controlled trial of fecal occult blood testing (17) and a case-control study of sigmoidoscopy (18) both find a protective effect. Causation is particularly supported when studies using several different research designs all lead to the same result, because studies using the same design can all make the same mistake.

It is often the case that different studies produce different results. Lack of consistency does not necessarily mean that the results of a particular study are invalid. One good study should outweigh several poor ones.

Biologic Plausibility

Whether the assertion of cause and effect is consistent with our knowledge of the mechanisms of disease as they are currently understood is often given considerable weight when assessing causation. When we have absolutely no idea how an association might have arisen, we tend to be skeptical that the association is real. Such skepticism often serves us well. For example, the substance Laetrile was touted as a cure for cancer in the early 1980s. However, the scientific community was not convinced, because they could think of no biologic reason why an extract of apricot pits not chemically related to compounds with known anticancer activity should be effective against cancer cells. To nail down the issue, Laetrile was finally submitted to a randomized controlled trial in which it was shown that the substance was, in fact, without activity against the cancers studied (19).

It is important to remember, however, that what is considered biologically plausible depends on the state of medical knowledge at the time. In Meig's day, contagious diseases were biologically implausible. Today, a biologically plausible mechanism for puerperal sepsis, the effects of streptococcal infection, has made it easier for us to accept Holmes's observations.

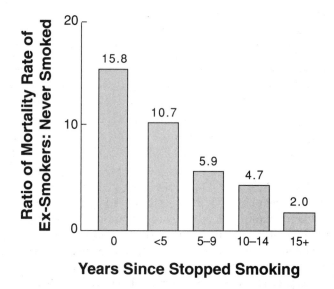

Figure 11.9. Reversible association: declining mortality from lung cancer in ex-cigarette smokers. The data exclude people who stopped smoking after getting cancer. (Drawn from Doll R, Petro R. Mortality in relation to smoking: 20 years' observations on male British doctors. Br Med J 1976;2:1525–1536.)

On the other hand, the mechanism by which acupuncture causes anesthesia is far less clear. To many scientists in the Western world, the suggestion that anesthesia is caused by sticking needles into the body and twirling them seems biologically implausible, and so they do not believe in the effectiveness of acupuncture.

In sum, biologic plausibility, when present, strengthens the case for causation. When it is absent, other evidence for causation should be sought. If the other evidence is strong, the lack of biologic plausibility may indicate the limitations of medical knowledge, rather than the lack of a causal association.

Specificity

Specificity—one cause, one effect—is more often found for acute infectious diseases (such as poliomyelitis and tetanus) and for inborn errors of metabolism (such as gout, ochronosis, and familial hypercholesterolemia). As we pointed out, for chronic, degenerative diseases there are often many causes for the same effect or many effects from the same cause. Lung cancer is caused by cigarette smoking, asbestos, and radiation. Cigarettes cause not only lung cancer but also bronchitis, peptic ulcer disease, periodontal disease, and wrinkled skin. The presence of specificity is strong evidence for cause, but the absence of specificity is weak evidence against a cause-and-effect relationship.

Analogy

The argument for a cause-and-effect relationship is strengthened if there are examples of well-established causes that are analogous to the one in question. Thus if we know that a slow virus can cause a chronic, degenerative central nervous system disease (subacute sclerosing panencephalitis), it is easier to accept that another virus might cause degeneration of the immunologic system (acquired immunodeficiency syndrome). In general, however, analogy is weak evidence for cause.

Weighing the Evidence

Most of this chapter has been a discussion of what to look for in individual studies when considering the possibility of a causal relationship. But, when deciding about cause, one must consider all the available evidence, from all available studies. After examining the pattern of evidence, the case for causality can be strengthened or eroded. This calls for a good deal of judgment, especially when the evidence from different studies is conflicting. In such cases, clinicians must decide where the weight of the evidence lies.

Figure 11.10 summarizes the different types of evidence for and against cause, depending on the research design, and features that strengthen or

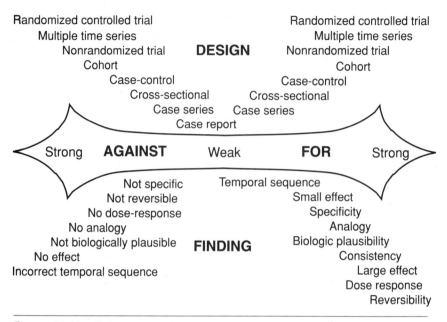

Figure 11.10. Relative strength of evidence for and against a causal effect. Note that with study designs, except for case reports and time series, the strength of evidence *for* a causal relationship is a mirror image of that *against*. With findings, evidence *for* a causal effect does not mirror evidence *against* an effect.

weaken the evidence for cause. The figure roughly indicates relative strengths in helping to establish or discard a causal hypothesis. Thus a carefully done cohort study showing a strong association and a dose-response relationship is strong evidence for cause, while a cross-sectional study finding no effect is weak evidence against cause.

Summary

Cause-and-effect relationships underlie diagnostic, preventive, and therapeutic activities in clinical medicine.

Diseases usually have many causes, although occasionally one might predominate. Often, several causes interact with one another in such a way that the risk of disease is more than would be expected by simply combining the effects of the individual causes taken separately. In other cases, the presence of a third variable, an effect modifier, modifies the strength of a cause-and-effect relationship between two variables.

Causes of disease can be proximal pathogenetic mechanisms or more remote genetic, environmental, or behavioral factors. Medical interventions to prevent or reverse disease can occur at any place in the development of disease, from remote origins to proximal mechanisms.

The case for causation is usually built over time with several different studies. It rests primarily on the strength of the research designs used to establish it. Because we rarely have the opportunity to establish cause using randomized controlled trials, observational studies are necessary. Some studies of populations (time series and multiple time series studies) may suggest causal relationships when a given exposure of groups of people is followed by a given effect.

Features that strengthen the argument for a cause-and-effect relationship include an appropriate temporal relationship, a strong association between purported cause and effect, the existence of a dose-response relationship, a fall in risk when the purported cause is removed, and consistent results among several studies. Biologic plausibility and coherence with known facts are other features that argue for a causal relationship.

REFERENCES

1. Holmes OW. On the contagiousness of puerperal fever. Med Classics 1936;1:207–268. [Originally published 1843.]
2. Webster's ninth new collegiate dictionary. Springfield, MA: Merriam-Webster, 1991.
3. MacMahon B, Pugh TF. Epidemiology: principles and methods. Boston: Little, Brown & Co., 1970.
4. Cantwell MF, Snider DE, Cauthen GM, Onorato IM. Epidemiology of tuberculosis in the United States, 1985 through 1992. JAMA 1994;272:535–539.
5. Weis SE, et al. The effect of directly observed therapy on the rates of drug resistance and relapse in tuberculosis. N Eng J Med 1994;330:1179–1184.
6. Goldman L. Analyzing the decline in the CAD death rate. Hosp Pract 1988;23(2):109–117.
7. Kannel WB. Preventive cardiology. Postgrad Med 1977;61:74–85.
8. Siscovick DS, et al. Diuretic therapy for hypertension and the risk of primary cardiac arrest. N Eng J Med 1994;330:1852–1857.
9. O'Conner GT, Morton JR, Diehl MJ, Olmstead EM, Coffin LH, Levy DG. Differences between men and women in hospital mortality associated with coronary artery bypass graft surgery. Circulation 1993;88(1):2104–2110.
10. St. Leger AS, Cochrane AL, Moore F. Factors associated with cardiac mortality in developed countries with particular reference to the consumption of wine. Lancet 1979;1:1017–1020.
11. Pear SM, Williamson TH, Bettin KM, Gerding DN, Galgian JN. Decrease in nosocomial *Clostridium* difficile-associated diarrhea by restricting clindamycin use. Ann Intern Med 1994;120:272–277.
12. Cervical Cancer Screening Programs. I. Epidemiology and natural history of carcinoma of the cervix. Can Med Assoc J 1976;114:1003–1033.
13. Bradford-Hill AB. The environment and disease: association or causation? Proc R Soc Med 1965;58:295–300.
14. Kuller L, Wing R. Weight loss and mortality. Ann Intern Med 1993;119:630–632.
15. Centers for Disease Control. Highlights of the surgeon general's report on smoking and health. MMWR 1979;28:1–11.
16. Beasley RP, Lin CC, Hwang LY, Chien CS. Hepatocellular carcinoma and hepatitis B virus. Lancet 1981;2:1129–1133.
17. Mandel JS, et al. Reducing mortality from colorectal cancer by screening for fecal occult blood. N Engl J Med 1993;328:1365–1371.

18. Selby JV, Friedman GD, Quesenberry CP, Weiss NS. A case-control study of screening sigmoidoscopy and mortality from colorectal cancer. N Engl J Med 1992;326:653–657.
19. Moertel CG, et al. A clinical trial of amygdalin (laetrile) in the treatment of human cancer. N Engl J Med 1982;306:201–206.

SUGGESTED READINGS

Buck C. Popper's philosophy for epidemiologists. Int J Epidemiol 1975;4:159–168
Chalmers AF. What Is this Thing Called Science? 2nd ed. New York: University of Queensland Press, 1982.
Department of Clinical Epidemiology and Biostatistics, McMaster University Health Sciences Centre. How to read clinical journals. IV: To determine etiology or causation. Can Med Assoc J 1981;124:985–990.
Rothman KJ (ed). Causal inference. Chestnut Hill, MA: Epidemiology Resources, 1988.

12

SUMMING UP

Where is the knowledge we have lost in information?
T. S. Eliot, "The Rock"

The usefulness of clinical research depends on its scientific credibility—its believability to thoughtful, unbiased scientists—and its relevance to the problems faced by clinicians and their patients. Both clinicians, who base their decisions on the medical literature, and researchers, who create it, need to understand what adds to and subtracts from the strength of scientific research.

To judge scientific credibility, readers must take an active role. They must decide what they want to discover from the medical literature and then see if the information is present and meets their standards of scientific credibility. By just reading passively, without considering the basic scientific principles systematically and in advance, they will be less likely to notice shortcomings and more likely to be misled.

This chapter describes how the methodologic principles discussed in previous chapters can be applied by busy clinicians to the lifelong task of trying to practice evidence-based medicine. First, we discuss how research articles pertaining to a given clinical question are identified and how their numbers can be reduced to manageable proportions without sacrificing needed information. Next, we summarize basic rules for judging the strength of individual articles; that section deals with concepts that have been discussed throughout the book. Third, we consider how the many articles on a given research question, as a group, are summarized to discover where the best available estimate of the truth lies. It is on this estimate that clinicians must base their clinical decisions until better information becomes available. Throughout the chapter we consider how these steps—article identification, study evaluation, and evidence synthesis—relate to strategies for keeping abreast of the literature throughout one's life as a clinician.

Whatever the strength of the best available evidence, clinicians must use it as a basis for action—sometimes rather bold action—yet regard it as fallible and subject to revision. One scholar (1) has distinguished between "decisions" and "conclusions." We decide something is true if we will act as if it is so, for the present, until better information comes along. Conclusions, on the other hand, are settled issues and are expected to be more durable. Clinicians are mainly concerned with decisions. The integrity of the scientific enterprise rests on the willingness of its participants to engage in open-minded, well-informed arguments for and against a current view of the truth, to accept new evidence, and to change their minds.

Approaches to Reading the Literature

Clinicians examine the medical literature from different perspectives, depending on their purpose. They browse to see what is interesting, they read articles of clinical interest to keep up, they look up the answers to specific clinical questions, and they systematically review the literature about a clinical issue to develop or change a clinical policy. We mainly deal with the full review of the literature. We understand that clinicians rarely have the time to do a full-blown review of existing information. However, if they understand the basic principles by which literature searches are done, they are in a better position to identify credible articles efficiently and judge the results for themselves when they browse, keep up, or look up information.

WHICH ARTICLES ARE IMPORTANT FOR CLINICAL DECISION MAKING?

All articles are not equally important for clinical decision making. Thoughtful clinicians must find and value the soundest articles in the face of an almost overwhelming body of available information.

Figure 12.1 summarizes an approach to distinguishing articles of fundamental importance to clinical decision making from those that are not. Many articles—reviews, teaching articles, editorials—are written to describe what is generally believed to be true but are not themselves reports of original research aimed at establishing that truth. These articles are a convenient source of summary information, but they are interpretations of the true knowledge base and are not independent contributions to it. Moreover, they are usually written by people with an established point of view, so that there is the potential for bias.

> *Example* How well do review articles and textbook chapters summarize the available body of scientific evidence about a clinical question? Investigators produced estimates of the effectiveness of various interventions to reduce morbidity and mortality from myocardial infarction (MI) by performing meta-analyses (described later in this chapter) of randomized clinical trials (RCTs) (2). The estimates were compared with expert recommendations published at the same point in time in review articles and textbook chapters. They found that "expert opinion" generally lagged behind the cumulative

Contribution to Answering
the Clinical Question

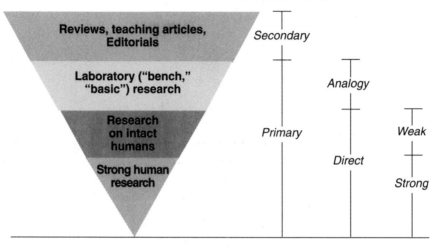

Figure 12.1. The literature on a research question: the relative value of various kinds of articles for answering a clinical question.

evidence by several years and not infrequently disagreed with it. For example, by 1980 there were 12 RCTs in the literature that had examined the efficacy of prophylactic lidocaine in the treatment of acute MI. Essentially, all showed that treatment with lidocaine was no better and often worse than placebo, yet the majority of review articles and chapters published during the 1980s continued to recommend routine or selective use of lidocaine.

Other articles describe original research done in laboratories for the purpose of understanding the biology of disease. These studies provide the richest source of hypotheses about health and disease. Yet, "bench" research cannot, in itself, establish with certainty what will happen in humans, because phenomena in actual patients, who are complex organisms in a similarly complex physical and social environment, involve variables that have been deliberately excluded from laboratory experiments.

Research involving intact humans and intended to guide clinical decision making ("clinical research") is, of course, conducted with varying degrees of scientific rigor. Even by crude standards, most studies are relatively weak. For example, a recent review of the methods of clinical studies in three surgical journals revealed that more than 80% had no comparison group, much less a randomized control group (3).

Throughout this book we have argued that the validity of clinical research depends on the strength of its methods (internal validity) and the extent to which it applies to a particular clinical setting (generalizability).

If this is so, a few good articles are more valuable than many weak or inappropriate ones. Thus the overall conclusion from the medical literature often depends on how a relatively few articles are interpreted. A review of the literature should involve selecting these articles carefully, identifying their scientific strengths and weaknesses, and synthesizing the evidence when their conclusions differ.

FINDING USEFUL ARTICLES

When systematically reviewing the literature, the first task is to locate articles that may be useful. This is most challenging when reviewing the literature, where it is first necessary to sort through a large number of titles, often thousands, to find the small number of articles that are useful. The objective is to reduce the literature to manageable proportions without missing important articles. The task can be intimidating and time-consuming. We describe a plan of attack, starting first with the full review of the literature.

The first step is to develop a set of criteria for screening titles to select articles that may be relevant while excluding a much larger number that clearly are not. The criteria should provide a sensitive test for the articles that one hopes to find in the same sense as a screening test should be sensitive for a disease, i.e., few useful articles should be missed. Initially, specificity can be sacrificed to achieve sensitivity, with the understanding that it will be necessary to evaluate many "false-positive" articles in more detail for each one that meets the final criteria. Often a useful screening algorithm is defined by the joint occurrence of a few key words in the title, e.g., *sarcoidosis, pulmonary,* and *corticosteroid* or *cancer, pancreatic,* and *diagnosis.*

Second, the screening criteria are applied to a list of journal titles, generally the list maintained by the National Library of Medicine, MEDLINE. Although available in bound volumes, many clinicians are currently accessing the medical literature electronically via modem, CD-ROM, or other computer-based systems. Because computer searching usually misses some important articles, one should also identify articles from other sources of titles such as recent review articles, other articles on the same topic, textbooks, and suggestions from experts in the field. The result of this search is a large number of titles, some of which represent relevant articles and many of which do not.

Third, one must apply specific criteria to identify the articles that are actually appropriate for the question at hand. Three kinds of criteria are often used:

• Does the article address the specific clinical question that was the reason for the search in the first place?

- Does the article represent original research, not secondary information or opinion?
- Is the research based on relatively strong methods?

Many inappropriate articles can be excluded by examination of the full title. Often, however, more information is required, and the abstract serves this purpose well. Perusal of abstracts should reveal to the reader whether a study of treatment used a comparison group and random allocation, a study of prognosis was on an inception cohort, whether a study has sufficient statistical power or precision, and so on.

Structured abstracts (4), which have been adopted by many of the leading medical journals, provide a better opportunity to judge potentially useful articles. The structured abstract summarizes in outline format those elements of a study—the research question, study design, setting, patients, interventions, measurements, results, and conclusions—required to distinguish valid and informative studies from the larger number that are not original or are inadequately rigorous.

Finally, one must actually look at the articles that remain to see which meet the final criteria. By this time, the number of articles should have been reduced enough that the task is feasible. Figure 12.2 summarizes these steps and illustrates the search process for a specific question: the outcome of total knee replacement (5).

If there is not sufficient time for a full, broadly based search for articles or the reader is browsing or trying to stay abreast of important developments, the early steps of this process must be abbreviated. One can examine only those journals that publish original research with high methodologic standards. However, this is an insensitive strategy: one would have to examine at least 11 of the world's best journals just to find 80% of the best articles on a question (6).

Another approach, is to have the screening of articles done by others. One would want them to be experts in both clinical medicine and clinical research methods, to examine all of the world's articles, and to make their criteria for inclusion explicit. The journal *ACP Journal Club* presents structured abstracts for the scientifically strong, clinically relevant original research in internal medicine, selected by explicit criteria published in each issue. The results of selection in this way are powerful: in 1993, there were more than 6 million articles published in clinical journals, of which about 350—a manageable number—met the criteria. Another option, the Cochrane Collaboration, is being developed. Expert groups from throughout the world are working together to select the best studies of clinical interventions, summarize them in a standard form, disseminate the information electronically, correct the database when errors are found, and keep it up

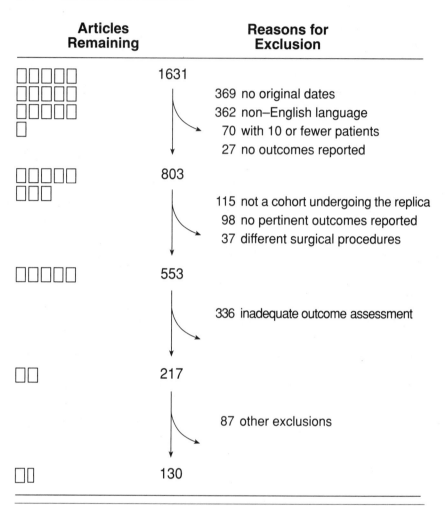

Articles Remaining	Reasons for Exclusion

1631

369 no original dates
362 non–English language
70 with 10 or fewer patients
27 no outcomes reported

803

115 not a cohort undergoing the replica
98 no pertinent outcomes reported
37 different surgical procedures

553

336 inadequate outcome assessment

217

87 other exclusions

130

Figure 12.2. Literature search: identifying the few most important articles from the medical literature as a whole. (Callahan CM, Drake BG, Heck DA, Dittus RS. Patient outcome following tricompartmental total knee replacement. JAMA 1994;271:1349–1357.)

to date. The results, at least for some clinical questions, should be available in the mid-1990s.

Judging Individual Articles

Once individual articles of interest have been identified, the next task is to evaluate the quality of the evidence they contain. The approach uses the scientific principles described in this book.

We have outlined basic criteria for the scientific credibility of specific research designs in the appendix to this chapter. We summarized a set of questions that should be asked of most studies—by investigators and readers alike. They concern the nature of the research question, the generalizability and clinical usefulness of the results, and two processes that can affect internal validity: bias and chance. We considered ground rules for studies of diagnosis, frequency, prognosis, treatment, and cause. The appendix describes basic issues that should be considered when deciding whether an article might be sufficiently strong to be useful in a literature review and in setting criteria to assign weights to articles when preparing a synthesis of the results of several articles.

DOES THE DESIGN FIT THE QUESTION?

One cannot speak of "good" or "bad" research designs in general without reference to the question they are intended to answer. Many clinically oriented methodologic assessment schemes give lower grades to observational designs such as the prevalence survey. This may be justified if the clinical question concerns preventive or therapeutic interventions, but inappropriate if considering studies of diagnostic tests. Table 12.1 matches clinical questions to the best research designs used to answer them. The table is meant to offer a guideline; it should not preclude creative but scientifically sound approaches other than those listed. For example, the best available evidence that periodic screening sigmoidoscopy may reduce deaths from colorectal cancer came from a rigorous case-control study (7). Because of the large numbers of patients and lengthy follow-up period required to test the efficacy of sigmoidoscopy in a randomized trial, this may be the only form of evidence available for some time.

Table 12.1
Matching the Strongest Research Designs to Clinical Questions

Question	Design
Diagnosis	Prevalence
Prevalence	Prevalence
Incidence	Cohort
Risk	Cohort
	Case control
Prognosis	Cohort
Treatment	Clinical trial
Prevention	Clinical trial
Cause	Cohort
	Case control

Table 12.2
Characteristics of a Study That Determine Whether It Can Test or Only Raise Hypotheses

Characteristic	Hypothesis Raising	Hypothesis Testing
Design	Weak	Strong
Hypotheses	None (or after data collected and analysed)	Stated before study begun
Comparisons	Many	Few
p-value	Large	Small
Results confirmed on separate data set	No	Yes

RAISING OR TESTING A HYPOTHESIS

The conclusions of an individual piece of research fall on a spectrum of believability according to the decisiveness of the scientific strategy used (see Chapter 11). At one end of the spectrum are reports that only suggest relationships, albeit potentially useful ones, without putting these ideas to the test. Most case reports serve this function. The conclusions of these studies are tentative; many are later refuted. At the other end of the spectrum are studies—e.g., large randomized controlled trials—that have put ideas to a rigorous test. Conclusions from these studies are more definitive. Most studies fall between these extremes.

A priori hypotheses are important. Without them, false-positive findings can make their way into the literature in the following way. Suppose one examines a large number of variables in a data set none of which is associated with any of the others in nature. As discussed in Chapter 9, if a large number of associations between variables are examined, some of them will be extreme enough to appear "real," even though the associations are only by chance. At a conventional level of statistical significance, $p < 0.05$, about 1 in 20 such comparisons will be statistically significant, by definition. Of course, the observed associations are "real" for the particular data set at hand—but not necessarily in the population—because the current sample may misrepresent all such samples from the population of interest.

Now suppose that one of these comparisons is selected out of the larger set of all possible comparisons and given special emphasis, perhaps because it fits well with existing biomedical theories. Suppose the other comparisons are minimized in the final report. Then the association, taken out of context, can appear very important. This process—random (chance) occurrence of associations followed by biased selection of interesting ones—is not unusual in published research.

There are several clues that signal the degree to which a given study is hypothesis testing rather than hypothesis raising (Table 12.2).

The first, a strong research design, is not a strictly separate factor from the others. Making hypotheses in advance and limiting the number of comparisons examined reduce the number of apparently "significant" comparisons that emerge from a study. The exploration for effects in various subgroups of a larger study population is a common analytic strategy that may result in chance or spurious associations. When hypotheses made in advance, a priori hypotheses, are confirmed, one can place more confidence in the findings. Alternatively, investigators can simply limit the number of comparisons made after the fact, so that there is less chance of false-positive findings for the study as a whole. Or they can insist on a particularly small p value before ruling out the role of chance in explaining particular findings.

Another strategy to protect against the acceptance of spurious or chance associations is to raise hypotheses on one set of data and test them on a separate one (Fig. 12.3). The availability of large data sets and statistical computer software makes it relatively easy for the analysis to include multiple variables, considered either separately or together in models. The analysis of multiple variables should be viewed as raising hypotheses, as the investigators rarely specify in advance what the model will find, much less the weight given to each finding. If the data set is large enough, it can be divided randomly in half, with one half being used to develop the model and the second half used to confirm it. Or it can be tested in a different setting. This latter process is illustrated in the following example.

> *Example* Investigators developed an index, including seven physical signs, for predicting the early recurrence of acute asthma after discharge from an emergency department (8). Among 205 patients at the investigators' medical center, patients from whom the index was developed, the index had a sensitivity of 95% and a specificity of 97%. The results were so striking that the index began to be put into clinical practice elsewhere.
>
> Later, two other groups of investigators independently tested the index in other settings (9,10). The results were disappointing. The sensitivity and specificity were 40% and 71%, respectively, in one study, and 18.1% and 82.4% in the other.

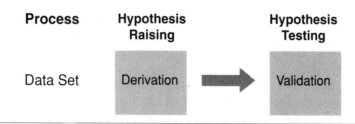

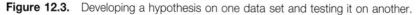

Figure 12.3. Developing a hypothesis on one data set and testing it on another.

These studies illustrate the dangers of placing too much confidence in a relationship that has been suggested in one data set but not tested in another, independent one. There are several possible reasons for the difference in performance. Patients in the original sample might have been systematically different, the index might have been applied differently, or chance might have resulted in unusual findings in the initial study.

Whatever the strategies used to increase the hypothesis-testing character of a study, it is the author's responsibility to make it clear where a particular study stands on the hypotheses-raising, hypothesis-testing spectrum and why. The readers' task is to seek out this information or reconstruct it, if it is not apparent. However, one should not eschew studies that mainly raise hypotheses; they are important, just not definitive.

Summarizing the Results of Many Studies

The current state of knowledge on a question is usually decided by the pattern of results from all studies addressing the question, rather than by one definitive study. Until recently, the commonest way of establishing this pattern was by implicit judgment, i.e., opinion, without having stated in advance the ground rules by which the contributions of individual studies would be weighted. Judgments of this sort often take the form of a traditional ("narrative") review article by an expert in the relevant field or a consensus of scholars representing the many points of view that bear on a question, e.g., the National Institutes of Health's Consensus Development Conferences.

A variety of more structured methods of summarizing published research is now used. These methods have the advantage of making explicit the assumptions behind the relative weights given to the various studies. They also follow the scientific method more directly: setting criteria in advance, gathering data (in this case, the results of individual studies), analyzing the data, and allowing the conclusions to follow from the criteria and data.

The process of summing up the research on a question, using structured methods, is referred to as *meta-analysis*—literally, analysis of analysis—or *information synthesis*. This approach is particularly useful when there is one specific question and at least a few relatively strong studies with apparently different conclusions. The use of these methods has exploded in the last few years. MEDLINE listed nearly 2000 articles under the subject heading "meta-analysis" between 1990 and mid-1994.

There are three general steps in performing a meta-analysis. First is to identify the best articles from all possible articles, as described earlier in this chapter. Second is to evaluate each study according to how well it meets methodological criteria, which are decided on in advance. In some meta-analyses, this evaluation results in the assignment of an overall qual-

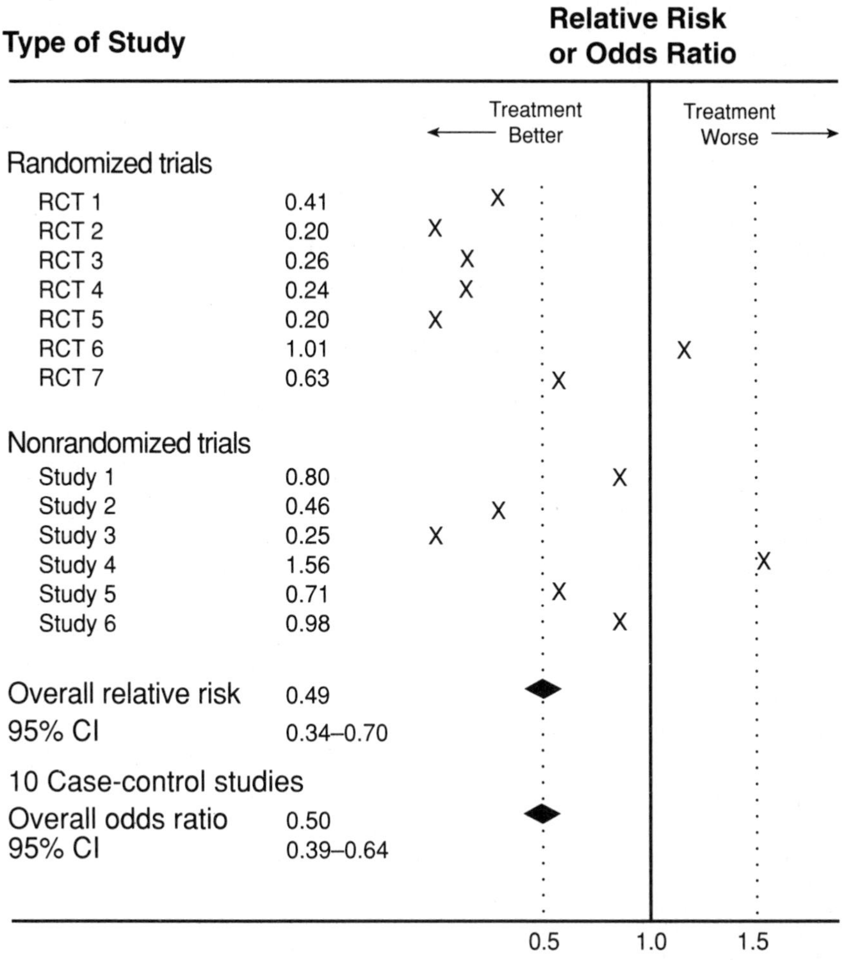

Type of Study — Relative Risk or Odds Ratio

Type of Study	Relative Risk or Odds Ratio
Randomized trials	
RCT 1	0.41
RCT 2	0.20
RCT 3	0.26
RCT 4	0.24
RCT 5	0.20
RCT 6	1.01
RCT 7	0.63
Nonrandomized trials	
Study 1	0.80
Study 2	0.46
Study 3	0.25
Study 4	1.56
Study 5	0.71
Study 6	0.98
Overall relative risk	0.49
95% CI	0.34–0.70
10 Case-control studies	
Overall odds ratio	0.50
95% CI	0.39–0.64

Axis (Treatment Better ← | → Treatment Worse): 0.5 1.0 1.5

Figure 12.4. Results of a meta-analysis of the effectiveness of BCG vaccination to prevent tuberculosis. *CI*, confidence interval. (Based on Colditz GA, Brewer TF, Berkey CS, Wilson ME, Burdick E, Fineberg HV, Mosteller F. Efficacy of BCG vaccine in the prevention of tuberculosis: meta-analysis of the published literature. JAMA 1994;271:698–702.)

ity score; in others, quality-related study characteristics of design, number and source of patients, and data collection methods are considered separately. The third step is to summarize, with numbers, the results of many studies to form, in effect, one large study with more statistical power than any of the individual studies alone. Each individual study is weighted by its sample size, i.e., large studies get more weight than ones with smaller numbers of patients. In addition, many meta-analyses also include the quality score as a weighting factor. Statistical methods, usually some form of regression analysis, are then used to estimate an overall effect measure, such as a relative risk or percentage reduction in mortality. Reports of meta-analyses include graphical displays of the results of the individual studies as well as the overall measure of effect.

Although meta-analysis has become the standard against which other approaches to literature synthesis are judged, there continues to be controversy about many of its elements, particularly the evaluation of quality and its inclusion in the overall assessment. But quality measures, while lumping disparate methodologic features in a single number, may help explain differences among studies.

> *Example* Although Bacille Calmette-Guerin (BCG) vaccine has been used to prevent tuberculosis for more than 50 years and is required in many countries, its efficacy is controversial. In part this is because the several large-scale clinical trials to evaluate BCG have reported conflicting results. An early meta-analysis compared the methods used in these trials to their results (11). The investigators found that the unbiased detection of tuberculosis in BCG and control groups was available only for the three trials reporting 75% or greater efficacy.

A more recent meta-analysis of the same question summarized the results of studies examining vaccine efficacy (12). Figure 12.4 shows the results of the seven randomized trials, six nonrandom trials, and the overall findings of the 10 case-control studies published as of 1994. Overall, in studies using each of the three designs, the risk of tuberculosis was found to be reduced by about half for those receiving the vaccination compared with those who did not. To help explain differences in observed magnitude of effect, the investigators developed overall scores for the quality of each study's methods. Using regression analysis, they found that better quality scores predicted findings of greater vaccine effect. The meta-analyses clearly establish the efficacy of BCG vaccine.

Often, however, there is no clear relationship between global quality ratings and their results. In this case, the meta-analysts must look at the specific methodologic features of studies to see why they are reaching disparate conclusions (13).

POOLING

Not uncommonly, the results of various individual studies are indecisive because each study describes too few patients or too few outcome events to have sufficient statistical power or precision. Consequently, estimates of rates from these studies are unstable, and each study's comparison of rates runs an unacceptably high risk of missing true effects (Type II error).

Pooling refers to the process of aggregating the data from several relatively small studies of the same question to form, in effect, one large one. It is permissible when it can be shown that the studies are sufficiently similar to each other (in patients, intervention and outcome measures) to treat them as if they are part of a single study. Pooling attempts to assemble enough observations to generate a precise overall estimate of effect, not to account for differences in conclusions among studies. The advantage of pooling is that it can result in adequate statistical power to detect meaningful differences, if they exist. Pooling is particularly useful when the disease and/or the outcome events of interest occur infrequently. Under these circumstances there are no other feasible ways to achieve statistical power.

> *Example*   There are many reports of peptic ulcer disease during corticosteroid therapy. Yet, it has been difficult to establish by means of observational studies whether corticosteroids cause ulcers, because many of the situations in which they are given—e.g., during stress and in conjunction with gastric-irritating drugs—may themselves predispose to peptic ulcer disease. Also, ulcers may be sought more diligently in patients receiving corticosteroids and go undetected in other patients.
>
> Randomized controlled trials are the best way to determine cause and effect. There have been many randomized trials in which corticosteroids were used to treat various conditions and peptic ulcer disease was a side effect. None of these studies was large enough in itself to test the corticosteroid/ulcer hypothesis. But together they provide an opportunity to examine the rate of rare event.
>
> In one review of 71 controlled trials of corticosteroids in which patients were randomized (or its equivalent) and peptic ulcer disease was considered, there were about 86 patients and 1 case of peptic ulcer disease per study; only 31 of the trials reported any patients with ulcers (14). The investigators pooled the results of these 71 trials to increase statistical power. In the pooled study, there were 6111 patients and about 80 ulcers. The rate of peptic ulcer disease was 1.8 in the corticosteroid group and 0.8 in the control group (relative risk, 2.3; 95% confidence interval, 1.4–3.7). The results were similar when examined separately according to the presence and absence of other risk factors; various doses, routes of administration, and duration of therapy; and whether the disease was suspected, defined as bleeding, or specifically diagnosed.
>
> Thus the combined results of many studies, each with relatively sound design but too small to answer the question, gave sufficient statistical power to detect risk.

Advocates of pooling point out that examination of the pattern of evidence, effectively summarized, can give new insights into the strengths and weaknesses of the evidence. For example, a single figure can show the number of strong studies, the point estimate and statistical precision of each study's observed effect size, the relationship between effect size and precision, and the point estimate and precision of their pooled effect (see Fig. 12.4).

Opponents of pooling argue that the ways in which patients, interventions, and outcomes were selected in the various studies are so dissimilar that it is not reasonable to combine them. "Splitters" are not as satisfied with pooling as "lumpers." Also, pooling deals only with statistical power. It does not correct for whatever biases existed in the designs of the various individual studies, nor can it be assumed that these biases cancel each other out when the studies are aggregated. In any case, meta-analyses only supplement and do not replace the insights gained by examining each of the best studies of a clinical question carefully.

Publication and Bias

Clinicians prefer good news, as does everyone else. Thus such words as *efficacy, predicting,* and *correlation* are the order of the day in journal titles. It is considerably less appealing to contemplate things that do not work. In fact, such observations are often considered failures. Researchers with the bad fortune to make such observations are likely to be advised by their friends, with gentle malice, to seek publication in the *Journal of Negative Results.*

It may be that our penchant for positive results leads to bias in the kinds of articles selected for publication in medical journals.

> *Example*   The final disposition of 285 studies that had been reviewed by an English Research Ethics Committee and brought to conclusion by the investigators was studied (15). Statistically significant results were found in 54% of studies, a nonsignificant trend in 16%, and null results in 30%. Of the studies with significant results, 85% were either published or presented as opposed to only 56% of studies with negative results (odds ratio, 4.54; 95% confidence interval, 2.4–8.6). Studies with null results were not of poorer quality, nor were they more likely to be unpublished because of editorial rejection.

Articles actually reaching publication are a biased sample of all research findings, tending to represent efforts to find causes, diagnostic tests, and treatments as being more effective than they actually are. For example, a meta-analysis of the relative effectiveness of single versus multiple drugs in ovarian cancer found a large survival advantage with multiple drugs in published data. When the investigator (16) added unpublished results, the difference disappeared. There is no reason to assert that biased judgments are made deliberately. Everyone does his or her part to put the "best" work forward, but publication is not a random process. There are forces favoring positive over negative results that are quite independent of the relative proportions of these results among all research projects undertaken. Readers should be aware of this bias lest they become unrealistically impressed with the many new and promising findings that appear in medical journals.

One way to avoid this bias is to give more credibility to large studies than to small ones. Most large studies, having required great effort and expense in their execution, will be published regardless of whether they have a positive or negative finding. Smaller studies, on the other hand, require less investment and so are more easily discarded in the selection process.

Different Answers: The Same Questions?

Until now, we have emphasized how studies can come to different conclusions because they have different methods, better for some than for others. But there is an alternative explanation: The research questions, although superficially the same, may actually be fundamentally different. Rather than one or the other study being misleading, both might be right. It may be that human biology, not research methods, accounts for the difference.

> *Example* Several authors (17,18) have performed meta-analyses assessing the effectiveness of drug treatment for hypertension. Early trials demonstrated substantial and statistically significant reductions in strokes but smaller and often not statistically significant reductions in coronary heart disease (CHD) (Fig. 12.5). The confidence interval for the pooled relative risk for CHD across all trials includes 1.
>
> More recent trials have focused on or at least included older adults. These newer trials, also summarized in Figure 12.5, showed the same degree of risk reduction for stroke but larger and consistently significant reductions in the risk of coronary heart disease. While the larger effectiveness of treatment observed in more recent trials suggests that drug therapy for hypertension is more effective in older patients than was previously believed, these newer trials tended to use diuretics and beta-blockers, the principal drugs in the trials, in lower doses, This may also have contributed to the greater effect of treatment on CHD.

Studies of cause and effect that seem to be asking similar questions can in fact present different questions in at least four ways: The patients, interventions, follow-up, and end results may not be the same. Differences among studies in any one of these may be enough to give different results.

Other Sources of Information

Until now the main source of information we have considered is journal articles reporting original research and meta-analyses based on them. What about other sources of information?

Textbooks are convenient and trustworthy for reporting well-established facts. But they have the disadvantage of being out of date (as much as 1 year old at time of publication) and reflecting the opinions of single authors, with little external review. Colleagues, especially those specialized in the area of the clinical questions, are also practical sources of informa-

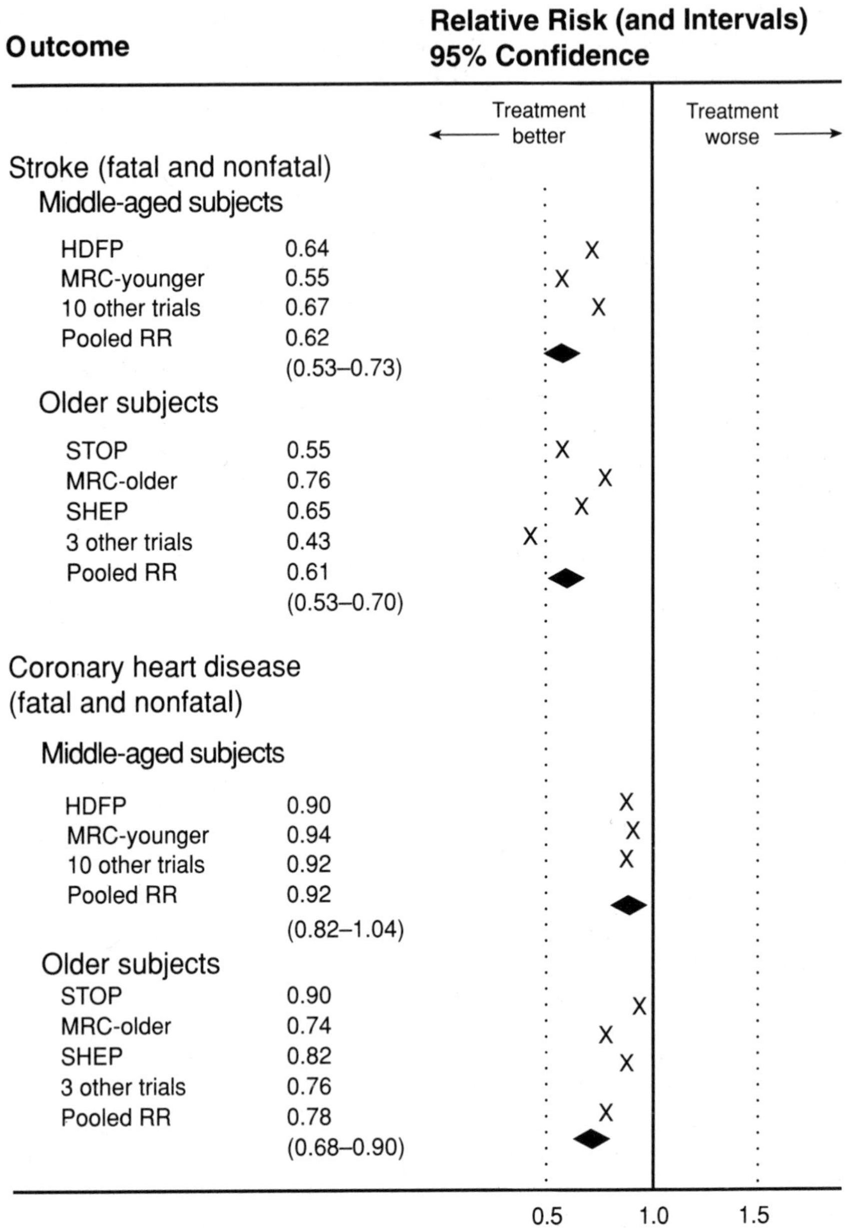

Outcome		Relative Risk (and Intervals) 95% Confidence

Stroke (fatal and nonfatal)
Middle-aged subjects

HDFP	0.64	X
MRC-younger	0.55	X
10 other trials	0.67	X
Pooled RR	0.62 (0.53–0.73)	◆

Older subjects

STOP	0.55	X
MRC-older	0.76	X
SHEP	0.65	X
3 other trials	0.43	X
Pooled RR	0.61 (0.53–0.70)	◆

Coronary heart disease (fatal and nonfatal)

Middle-aged subjects

HDFP	0.90	X
MRC-younger	0.94	X
10 other trials	0.92	X
Pooled RR	0.92 (0.82–1.04)	◆

Older subjects

STOP	0.90	X
MRC-older	0.74	X
SHEP	0.82	X
3 other trials	0.76	
Pooled RR	0.78 (0.68–0.90)	◆

0.5   1.0   1.5

Figure 12.5. Results of a meta-analysis of the efficacy of hypertension control on the risk of stroke and coronary heart disease. (Adapted from Cutler JA, Pstay BM, MacMahon S, Furberg CD. Public health issues in hypertension control. What has been learned from clinical trials? In: Laragh JH, Brenner BM, eds. Hypertension: physiology, diagnosis, and management. 2nd ed. New York: Raven Press, 1995.)

tion, but their opinions are only as good as the consultant, who may be biased by the beliefs and financial interests of his or her field. For example, it is natural for gastroenterologists to believe in endoscopy more than radiologic contrast studies and surgeons to believe in surgery over medical therapy.

A growing number of databases are complete, up to date, and widely available by telephone, fax, floppy disks, CD-ROM, and e-mail, the Internet, and compter bulletin board. Examples include a 24-hr telephone connection to the Centers for Disease Control and Prevention for information about disease prevention offered to those traveling to any part of the world; Toxline for information on poisonings; PDQ for current recommendation for cancer chemotherapy; and an array of databases on drugs, their toxicities, and adjustment of dose in renal failure. These databases contain information that is essential to the practice of medicine but are too infrequently needed and too extensive for clinicians to carry around in their heads. Clinicians should find ways to access them in their location. They should also use these databases with the lessons of this book in mind: The data are only as good as the methods used to select them. Many of the databases, such as guidelines of the Agency for Health Care Policy and Research, the U.S. Preventive Services Task Force, and the American College of Physicians, are created by excellent methods and make the process clear. Some are the results of individuals or industries with conflict of interest, and they should be used with skepticism.

Clinical Guidelines

Throughout the book we have argued that clinical research provides the soundest grounds for establishing one's approach to clinical practice and making decisions about patients. The shift away from anecdote and personal experience has been called "evidence-based medicine" (19). An important element in evidence-based medicine is the translation of research findings into clear, unambiguous recommendations for clinicians. Practice guidelines are systematically developed statements to assist clinicians in deciding about appropriate health care for specific clinical problems (19). Their development and use are now commonplace in many organized medical settings. At their best, the validity of guidelines is established by including in the panel that prepares them people who represent all relevant aspects of the question (ranging from highly specialized researchers to clinicians, economists ,and patients) to cover all important aspects of the question and to balance, if not eliminate, the vested interests of any one or another participant. The best guidelines are based on research evidence, not just expert opinion, and so often use formal processes of literature review and synthesis, as described in this chapter (20).

Guidelines are meant to guide, not prescribe clinical judgment. There are good reasons not to follow guidelines in the care of some individual patients.

Do guidelines change physicians' behavior? A meta-analysis identified and summarized 59 published articles that evaluated the impact of explicit guidelines using more rigorous research designs—randomized trials, nonrandomized comparative trials, and interrupted time series designs (21). More than 90% of the studies demonstrated significant changes in care in accordance with the guidelines, and 9 out of the 11 studies examining patient outcomes showed improvements.

REFERENCES

1. Tukey JW. Conclusions and decisions. Technometrics 1960;2:423–433.
2. Antman EM, Lau J, Kupelnick B, Mosteller F, Chalmers TC. A comparison of results of meta-analyses of randomized trials and recommendations of clinical experts: treatment of myocardial infarction. JAMA 1992;268:240–248.
3. Soloman MJ, McLeod RS. Clinical studies in surgical journals—have we improved? Dis Colon Rectum 1993;36:43–48.
4. Haynes RB, Mulrow CD, Huth EJ, Altman DG, Gardner MJ. More informative abstracts revisited. Ann Intern Med 1990;113:69–75.
5. Callahan CM, Drake BG, Heck DA, Dittus RS. Patient outcome following tricompartmental total knee replacement. A meta-analysis. JAMA 1994;271:1349–1357.
6. Haynes RB. Where's the meat in clinical journals? [Editorial]. ACP J Club 1993;Nov–Dec:A22–A23. [Originally published in Ann Intern Med 1993;114(Suppl 1).]
7. Selby JV, Friedman GD, Quesenberry CP Jr, Weiss NS. A case control study of screening sigmoidoscopy and mortality from colorectal cancer. N Engl J Med 1992;326:653–657.
8. Fischl MA, Pitchenik A, Gardner LB. An index predicting relapse and need for hospitalization in patients with acute bronchial asthma. N Engl J Med 1981;305:783–789.
9. Rose CC, Murphy JG, Schwartz JS. Performance of an index predicting the response of patients with acute bronchial asthma to intensive emergency department treatment. N Engl J Med 1984;310:573–577.
10. Centor RM, Yarbrough B, Wood JP. Inability to predict relapse in acute asthma. N Engl J Med 1984;310:577–580.
11. Clemens JD, Chuong JH, Feinstein AR. The BCG controversy: a methodological and statistical reappraisal. JAMA 1983;249:2362.
12. Colditz GA, Brewer TF, Berkey CS, Wilson ME, Burdick E, Fineberg HV, Mosteller F. Efficacy of BCG vaccine in the prevention of tuberculosis: meta-analysis of the published literature. JAMA 1994;271:698–702.
13. Greenland S. A critical look at some popular meta-analytic methods [Invited Commentary]. Am J Epidemiol 1994;140:290–296.
14. Messer J, Reitman D, Sacks HS, Smith H Jr, Chalmers TC. Association of adrenocorticosteroid therapy and peptic-ulcer disease. N Engl J Med 1983;309:21–24.
15. Easterbrook PJ, Berlin JA, Gopalan R, Matthews DR. Publication bias in clinical research. Lancet 1991;337:867–872.
16. Simes RJ. Confronting publication bias: a cohort design for meta-analysis. Stat Med 1987;6:11–29.
17. Cutler JA, Psaty BM, MacMahon S, Furberg CD. Public health issues in hypertension control: what has been learned from clinical trials? In: Laragh JH, Brenner BM, eds. Hypertension: physiology, diagnosis, and management. 2nd ed. New York: Raven Press, 1995.

18. Hebert PR, Fiebach NH, Eberlein KA, Taylor JO, Hennekens CH. The community based randomized trials of pharmacological treatment of mild-to-moderate hypertension. Am J Epidemiol 1988;127:581–589.
19. Evidence based medicine working group. Evidence based medicine: a new approach to teaching the practice of medicine. JAMA 1992;268:2420–2425.
20. Hayward RSA, Wilson MC, Tunis SR, Bass EB, Rubin HR, Haynes RB. More informative abstracts of articles describing clinical practice guidelines. Ann Intern Med 1993;118:731–737.
21. Grimshaw JM, Russell IT. Effect of clinical guidelines on medical practice. A systematic review of rigorous evaluations. Lancet 1993;342:1317–1321.

SUGGESTED READING

Epidemiology Work Group of the Interagency Regulatory Liaison Group. Guidelines for documentation of epidemiologic studies. Am J Epidemiol 1981;114:609–713.
Goldschmidt PG. Information synthesis: a practical guide. Health Services Res 1986;21:215–237.
Haynes RB McKibbon KA, Fitzgerald D, Guyatt GH, Walker CJ, Sackett DL. How to keep up with the medical literature. 1: Why try to keep up and how to get started. Ann Intern Med 1986;105:149–153.
Haynes RB, McKibbon KA, Fitzgerald D, Guyatt GH, Walker CJ, Sackett DL. How to keep up with the medical literature. II: Deciding which journals to read regularly. Ann Intern Med 1986;105:309–312.
Haynes RB, McKibbon KA, Fitzgerald D, Guyatt GH, Walker CJ, Sackett DL. How to keep up with the medical literature. III: Expanding the number of journals you read regularly. Ann Intern Med 1986;105:474–478.
Haynes RB, McKibbon KA, Fitzgerald D, Guyatt GH, Walker CJ, Sackett DL. How to keep up with the medical literature. IV: Using the literature to solve clinical problems. Ann Intern Med 1986;105:636–640.
Haynes RB, McKibbon KA, Walker CJ, Mousseau J, Baker LM, Fitzgerald D, Guyatt G, Norman GR. Computer searching of the medical literature: an evaluation of MEDLINE searching systems. Ann Intern Med 1985;103:812–816.
Irwig L, Tosteson AN, Gastonis C, Lau J, Colditz G, Chalmers TC, Mostellar F. Guidelines for meta-analyses evaluating diagnostic tests. Ann Intern Med 1994;120:667–676.
L'Abbe KA, Detsky AS, O'Rourke K. Meta-analysis in clinical research. Ann Intern Med 1987;107:224–233.
Light RJ, Pillmer DB. Summing up. The science of reviewing research. Cambridge, MA: Harvard University Press, 1984.
Mulrow CD. State of the science [The Medical Review Article]. Ann Intern Med 1987;106:485–488.
Thompson SG, Pocock SJ. Can meta-analyses be trusted? Lancet 1991;338:1127–1130.

APPENDIX 12.1. BASIC GUIDELINES FOR DETERMINING THE VALIDITY OF CLINICAL STUDIES

ALL STUDIES

1. What *kind of clinical question* is the research intended to answer?
   The research design should match the clinical question (see Table 12.1)
2. What *patients, variables, and outcomes* were studied?
   These determine the generalizability of the results.

3. How likely is it that the findings are the result of *bias?*
   Systematic differences between compared groups (e.g., in patients' characteristics, interventions, or risk factors; outcomes; or measurement methods) diminish internal validity.
4. How big is the effect?
   Clinical decisions depend on the magnitude (not just on the existance) of effect.
5. How likely is it that the findings occurred by *chance?*
   Clinicians need to know the range of values within which the true effect is likely to fall (confidence interval) or (less useful) how likely the observed effect is by chance alone (*p* value for "positive" results and power for "negative" results).

STUDIES OF DIAGNOSTIC TESTS

1. Is the *test clearly described* (including the point at which it is considered abnormal)?
   If the test result can take on a range of values, the performance varies according to the choice of cutoff point.
2. Is the true presence or absence of disease (*gold standard*) established for all patients?
   It is possible to know all important aspects of test performance only if there are data for all four cells of the 2 by 2 table.
3. Does the *spectrum of patients* with and without disease match the characteristics of patients for whom the test will be used?
   Sensitivity is often affected by the severity of disease and specificity by the characteristics of those in the study without the disease.
4. Is there an *unbiased* assessment of test and disease status?
   Bias can occur if the test result is determined with knowledge of disease status and vice versa.
5. Is *test performance* summarized by sensitivity and specificity or likelihood ratio?
   This information is needed to decide whether to use the test.
6. For tests with a range of values, how does *moving the cutoff point* affect test performance?
   The information conveyed by the test depends on the degree of abnormality.
7. If *predictive value* is reported, is it in relation to a clinically sensible prevalence?
   Predictive value depends on prevalence (as well as the sensitivity and specificity of the test). If people with and without the disease are chosen separately, without relation to the clinicaly occurring prevalence, the resulting predictive value has no clinical meaning.

PREVALENCE STUDIES

1. What are the criteria for being a *case?*
   Prevalence depends on what one calls a case.
2. In what *population* are the cases found?
   Prevalence depends on the group of people in which it is described.
3. Is prevalence described for an *unbiased sample* of the population?
   Prevalence for the sample estimates prevalence for the population to the extent that the sample is unbiased.

COHORT STUDIES

1. Are all members of the cohort:
   a. Entered at the beginning of follow-up (*inception cohort*)?
      Otherwise people who do unusually well or badly will not be counted in the result.
   b. *At risk* for developing the outcome?
      It makes no sense to describe how outcomes develop over time in people who already have the disease or cannot develop it.
   c. At a similar point (*zero time*) in the course of disease?
      Prognosis varies according to the point in the course of disease at which one begins counting outcome events.
2. Is there *complete follow-up* on all members?
   Drop-outs can bias the results if they on average have a better or worse course than those who remain in the study.
3. Are all members of the cohort *assessed for outcomes with the same intensity?*
   Otherwise differences in outcome rates might be from measurement bias, not true differences.
4. Are *comparisons unbiased?* (would members of the cohorts have the same outcome rate except for the variable of interest?)
   To attribute outcome to the factor of interest other determinants of outcome must occur equally in the groups compared.

RANDOMIZED TRIALS

1. Are the basic *guidelines for cohort studies* satisfied?
   Clinical trials are cohort studies
2. Were *patients randomly allocated* to treated and control groups?
   This is the only effective way to make a completely unbiased comparison of treatments.
3. Were patients, caregivers, and researchers unaware of the treatment group (*masked*) to which each patient belonged?
   Masking participants in a trial helps assure that they are unbiased.
4. Were *cointerventions* the same in both groups?
   Treating patients differently can destroy the comparability that was achieved by randomization.

5. Were results described according to the *treatment allocated or the treatment actually received?*
   If not all patients receive the treatment assigned to them there are two kinds of analyses with different objectives and scientific strengths. "Intention to treat" analyses are for management decisions and are of the randomly constituted groups. "Efficacy" analyses are to explain the effect of the intervention itself, are of the treatment actually received, and are a cohort study.

CASE-CONTROL STUDIES

1. Were cases entered at the *onset* of disease?
   Risk factors for prevalent cases may be related to onset or duration of disease.
2. Were *controls similar to cases* except for exposure?
   A valid estimate of relative risk depends on an unbiased comparison.
3. Were there similar and unbiased *efforts to detect exposure* in cases and controls?
   Biased measurement of exposure can increase or decrease the estimate of relative risk.

META-ANALYSES

1. Is *all relevant research* (both published and unpublished studies) found?
   The objective is to summarize the results of all completed research, not a biased sample of it.
2. Does the meta-analysis include *only scientifically strong studies* (those with a low probability of bias)?
   The objective is to summarize the most credible evidence.
3. If a summary estimate of effect is calculated
   a. Are the studies *homogeneous* (are patients, interventions, and outcomes similar)?
      It is inappropriate to seek a single, overall measure of effect from inherently dissimilar studies.
   b. Are the studies *weighted* by their size?
      Larger (more precise) studies deserve more weight than smaller (less precise) ones.
4. Are study *quality and result related?*
   Better studies are more believable.

INDEX

Page numbers in *italics* denote figures; those followed by a "t" denote tables.